Wonderful Wavicle Work

How to Create Whatever You Need With Unconditional Love

Rory Goff

10/1/15

FOR KAREN,
A TRUE BRANCH
OF THE TREE OF
LIFE!
LOVE, LIGHT, &
LAUGHTER ALWAYS,
Rory

Disclaimer: Rory Goff is a spiritual teacher, and imparts knowledge and techniques which are spiritual only. None of his teachings or techniques is intended to be used as a substitute for any services provided by mental, emotional, or physical health professionals, or by professional financial advisors.

Table of Contents

Chapter One

What is Wavicle Work?

I want to show you a simple, effective technique that has radically improved my life and the lives of many others I have been privileged to know. Apparently both age-old and brand-new, the practice seems to have been lost and rediscovered many times through history. I cannot say with absolute certainty that it is for everyone, but if you are reading this, it might well be for you.

I call this technique *Wavicle Work* (or WW). Physicists invented the term *wavicle* when they discovered that everything in creation has the properties of infinitely-flowing, interconnected waves of energy and separate, discrete particles of matter simultaneously: *Wave* plus *particle* equals *wavicle*. Wavicles are especially noticeable in light-radiation, and light symbolizes your own consciousness. Just like light, your consciousness arises and appears both as a thought-*wave* and as an I-*particle*. And just as the *speed of light squared* is the constant intermediary and conversion factor between energy and matter, so your *consciousness aware of itself* is the constant intermediary and conversion factor between your spirit and your body. The art of enhancing your consciousness of your everyday reality is light-work, or Wavicle Work.

Whether it arises in your consciousness as a thought, feeling, or perception, every wavicle is simply your own indescribable Wholeness collapsed into a thought-wave or an I-point, creating a unique space-time story in your awareness. Each of your wavicles, whether internal or external, is one of your creations, a light-being, one of your children. You could call it an angel or a demon, depending on whether it is experiencing and giving you happiness or suffering at this moment, but in actuality it is simply part of your own Wholeness, wanting to come home.

Any painful thought or emotion you feel like "I want..." or "I need...." is a suffering wavicle who needs your attention, needs some Wavicle Work. A wavicle may appear abstract or external, but with a few deep breaths you can easily trace the thought or emotion back to a conscious tension-flow or attention-point in the body of your awareness. Wavicle Work is an easy, natural, seven-step process which reminds you that you are already Awake and naturally unbound. It shows you how to *localize* your painful wavicle by disidentifying yourself from a painful internal thought, or by taking responsibility for a painful external situation. Then, whether inner or outer, you may serve as its Witness and its personal Creator. Treating it as your divine child, you love it unconditionally and give it the fulfillment of whatever it truly needs: not with something in the outer world but here and now, on your inner finest, subtlest feeling level. You welcome it home into a new reality of Heaven on Earth.

When you have integrated all of the inevitable objections to your new reality from it and your other wavicles, you as Creator are done, and your reality or creation has shifted. Your thought-wavicles or creatures are essentially your subtle senses, so whatever you do for your creatures, your "little children," you do for yourself. As your subtle senses, wavicles take your innermost thoughts and translate them into your concrete exterior reality. Remind them of their divine nature and welcome them into Paradise on Earth, and you do the same for yourself.

As an internal thought-wavicle first arises, you generally identify with it, losing yourself in it, believing that its "I AM" is the totality of your own "I AM." This is perhaps because in the whole Universe, there is really only one "I AM," which has apparently multiplied itself endlessly in order to create. Entertaining a thought-wave or a bound sense of self is natural — it is through these creature-selves that your unbounded Creator-self knows and enjoys your space-time creation — but identifying completely with any wavicle eventually brings discomfort and suffering as you forget your infinite and eternal nature and come to believe in separation, limitation, and ignorance.

2

If you are identifying with a specific internal thought-wavicle, you tend to perceive all your other wavicles as outside of you and unrelated to you. If any wavicle, internal or external, is causing you suffering, it is because you are rejecting it as not-good, or not-God. *It is never the flavor of a wavicle which makes you suffer; it is always simply your rejection of it, or resistance to it.*

By rejecting it, you devilize or diabolize it – that is, cast it away from you. The words *devil* and *diabolic* come from the Greek *diaballein*, meaning "to throw across." As you are its source and its heavenly home, the wavicle then experiences rejection from its Creator and exile from heaven. It suffers, and then you suffer through it. Again, wavicles are essentially your subtle senses; what they feel, you feel.

There is absolutely nothing wrong with this process; it is a fundamental part of your creation and your healing. You grow by sending wavicles out of your Wholeness into the unknown, and then re-membering them. When you fully identify with any wavicle as separate from Wholeness, you are going to suffer, because that is not who you really are. The suffering is given by Grace, by the love of your own Wholeness, as a wake-up call.

The word *demon* comes from the Greek *daimon* meaning a deity, lesser god, or guiding spirit, so to *demonize* a wavicle should really mean only that you are recognizing that it is not your Wholeness, not who you really are. Eventually, you remember that you are not your suffering; that the wavicle you have been identifying with is, indeed, just a wavicle, only a *daimon*, not your Wholeness, and your first instinct is to name it and fully disidentify with it, to cast it out. Knowing you are no longer subject to your wavicle is a necessary step to full healing, but it is not yet full healing.

This is what the process of exorcism appears to have become – the naming and casting out of demons in the name of the Creator, in the name of Wholeness or Holiness. But "exorcism" comes from the Greek *exorkizein*, "to exorcise, or *to bind by oath.*" In English, the word *exorcise* originally simply meant "to call up" or "to conjure spirits," and the added meaning "to drive out" was not recorded until 1546. And the word *conjure* in Middle French meant "to plot or exorcise," from Latin *con* meaning "with" and *jurare* meaning "to swear." To *conjure* was "to band together with an oath." So both *conjure* and *exorcise* actually mean, "to cause to swear a binding oath" and "to band together:" that is, to bring into Wholeness, to integrate, to heal.

An *oath* is a solemn appeal to deity in witness of a truth or promise. As a wavicle you might avoid taking oaths, for you do not really know the ultimate truth, nor have any real control over creation, and it is wise not to bind yourself with promises you can't keep. The best way to "exorcise" or "conjure" is to *witness* your wavicle as its *Creator* and to bring it back into *truthful*, harmonious unity with you by *promising* to love it un-conditionally and meet its deepest needs utterly on your inner-most level of subtlest, finest feeling. When you do that for your wavicle, it willingly serves you in love and light and bliss.

Disidentifying with your suffering wavicle and remembering your fundamental Wholeness is the first half of your healing. The last half is bringing your wavicle into full identity with you as its Wholeness and Creator, converting it back from suffering demon into devoted angel. You do this best by meeting its sub-tlest needs from the understanding and unconditional love of Wholeness.

Though you may not currently experience or believe yourself to be the Creator of your entire universe, you are made in your Creator's image and likeness, which means that you are the co-creator of *your* reality. You do create your own thought-wavicles; they emerge from your consciousness, and those wav-icles include your beliefs and perceptions, which do determine your reality or universe. When you think unhappy thoughts, your day looks gloomy. When you think loving thoughts, your day is radiantly joyous. The better your relationship with your creature-wavicles, the better you as a creature will enjoy your relationship with your own Creator, for what you give to your creatures, you inevitably receive as a creature from the Creator of your universe, your own larger Self or infinite Wholeness.

As Wavicle Work heals your demons back into angels, you show them – and hence yourself – ever more abundant blessings of Heaven on Earth. The bodily integrity of your *Love* draws everything and everyone into a laser-like coherence of *Light* to ascend in joyous *Laughter* here and now, remembering there's only One of us.

The more repellent the demon or unpleasant quality you see, the greater the angelic gift it has to offer you when you integrate it in unconditional love. One of my favorite fairy tales speaks of the king who sends his three sons out into the world to seek their fortune. The older two sons spur their horses out across the castle drawbridge and soon encounter an old hag sitting in the middle of the road. Her rheumy eyes are as cold as the pale gray winter sky; she is clad in black rags and covered in mud; her bone-white, tangled hair looks like an osprey nest, and she smells of excrement. With a toothless grin, her mouth opens wide as an open sewer. She holds up her withered arms and screams, "Give us a kiss!" The two older sons give her one disgusted look and ride off into obscurity.

The youngest son leaves the castle on foot, but he too soon comes across the old hag. "Give us a kiss!" She screams. The lad gulps but politely says, "Yes, my lady!" And holding his breath he gingerly embraces and kisses her. To his shock he suddenly sees he has kissed a woman who is young, beautiful, and richly clad, with a fragrance of roses and jasmine and cinnamon. "I am the Land; I am your sovereignty," she smiles. "Because you were willing to embrace me in my ugliness, you now possess me in my beauty forever, my King!" This is the very essence of Wavicle Work, of using unconditional Love to enlighten your suffering demons into your blissful angels and best friends.

About nine years ago I encountered something like this fairy tale. I was suddenly struck by the *Matrix*-like nature of the physical world, by my consciousness being imprisoned forever in its sheer mechanistic determinism, in its overwhelmingly impersonal machine-like mortality.

My first instinct was to pull away in horror, but then I remembered Wavicle Work's lesson: the more repellent the demon, the greater the gift. So I figuratively held my breath, gave this imprisoning demon of death my full attention, and internally embraced it whole-heartedly, using the technique outlined in Chapter Two. And suddenly to my surprise the whole world had become my own body, and it was alive and on fire with indescribable *Love*!

And for the next week I remained in this blissful conflagration, physically overwhelmed with an intensely ecstatic, divine Love of the world. Through Wavicle Work's unconditional love, the horrifying demon had become one of the most beautiful angels I have ever known. But that is getting ahead of myself; here is how it all started:

First Wavicle-Work Experience: Awakening into Perfection

I have been practicing the Art of Wavicle Work for the past 32 years. After Transcendental Meditation and the TM-Sidhis program, Wavicle Work has been the single most important discovery in my life. After two years of an excruciating Dark Night of the Soul, of empty meaningless bleakness, I stumbled onto Wavicle Work in November 1982, when in a sudden moment of clarity I realized that my nine-year enlightenment search had been like a carrot on a stick. Enlightenment was forever ahead of me, just out of reach.

I had accumulated a great many enlightenment *experiences:* the birth of the impersonal Witness consciousness, the baptism of kundalini-energies and perception of celestial realms, the transfiguring golden unity with angels and nature and humans, but by definition, experiences came and went; everything had now died into a great Void and I was searching for something – *anything* – eternal and permanent. I didn't fully understand that I had been looking for Love in all the wrong places: inside of space-time, which is ever-changing.

Suddenly I realized that if what I sought was truly eternal and permanent, then it had to be here now and always. And if it was and always had been truly here now, then I must be overlooking it in favor of some imagined idea of what it was "supposed" to be. I saw that I needed to stop reaching for the carrot because it was attached to the stick of *not-this*: needed to stop believing completely in time and space, and even in evolution, in spiritual growth itself.

My next thought was, *"If everything I truly seek and need is already eternally present here and now, what is it I truly need in this moment?"* My insides lit up with a feeling of *"I'm glad you finally asked!"* At last I was asking what *I* needed, no longer trying to measure myself against someone else's criteria. *Self*-realization now became possible. What *did* I most need in this moment?

The answer that arose was simple but bold: *"Perfection!"* So Perfection must somehow already be here, now, even in this utter ordinariness and bleakness. I began to feel into that, and within the light of my awareness I immediately perceived a number of objections from within my body. *"But... but... if we have perfection, we will cease to exist, because we thrive on imperfection; we exist to correct things!"*

I found myself responding to these little I's, telling them, *"It's OK; you can live now, even in Perfection!"* A number of other objections arose and I answered them all, feeling down deeper and deeper into my body as it shook and wept.

Finally done, I opened my eyes and saw to my shock "I" had turned inside out: What I had thought was my deepest Self, inside, was now absolutely everywhere, and what I had thought was not-Self, outside, was now at the very core of my body, as if I had a hole through my middle. Inside I was Nothing; outside I was Everything.

Reality had awakened to Itself, or rather, I had ceased to overlay my beliefs on what *is*, the indescribable paradoxical perfection that has self-evidently always been here and now. Everything – that fire hydrant, Archangel Michael, the muck on the sidewalk – *everything* now was exactly the same perfect mind-stuff. Now my intellect was trying to make sense of this, trying to create a story to describe it, but it was like trying to pin down liquid mercury. Whatever I formulated, Reality immediately showed me it was also the opposite: *"Wow! This is so empty... no, it's full! It is obvious... no, it isn't obvious at all! It is permanent... no, it is evanescent! ... "* It – the Self -- is indeed subtler than the dualistic intellect, and is no-thing, and everything. It is simply Wholeness.

Wholeness whispered: *"This is Brahman; this is Nirvana; this is the Crucifixion.... You have resolved 51% of your karma, and no longer need reincarnate on Earth. You are free to leave now, if you wish, but you will continue to be born onto subtler and subtler planes, and you might wish to stay here, as you will be able to finish the remaining Work much faster here than there."*

That made some sense, but I still wasn't quite comfortable with the frozen crystalline perfection pervading everything. Later that day, a friend read to me from the Brahma Sutras, and the phrase *"Prana is Brahman"* brought my attention to *prana*, to the life-energy in my breath. Immediately, the crystalline "ice" warmed up into a dynamic dance of I-particles, tiny beings with whom I could interact. *They* still believed in space, time, and evolution. I saw that the remaining Work consisted entirely of attending to breath, putting my attention on these I-particles, and giving them whatever they needed: in short, Wavicle Work.

Second Wavicle-Work Experience: Surrendering via Particle Prayer into Infinite Abundance

A few days later, I wondered why, if the world was my co-creation as was now self-evident, was I still feeling the pinch of poverty? It was all clearly perfect as it was, but perhaps we could reshape that perfection into something even more perfect. For this I decided to imagine an all-powerful God in front of me – some One who was responsible for actually concretizing my world. Even if it was just a projection of my own conscious-ness, it would help to have someone to talk this out with.

I imagined a radiantly golden Being in front of me, and said po-litely, "Um... God?"

8

Nothing. There was no connection between us. *Well*, I thought, *let's get real here*. How did I really feel?

Wow. I was *angry!* I started to yell at God: "God *damn* it, God!" I yelled. "I am tired of being poor!" *Wham!* Suddenly there was a tunnel of Love connecting my heart to God's heart, and God became unquestionably real, fully present. *Hm! That's interesting!* I thought. *Truth is a carrier-wave of Love!*

This was new to me. If I had dared to express honest anger to my birth-father, he probably would have hit me. He was the only family member allowed to be angry; he had preferred a subservient politeness from his children, and that is what we had quickly learned to show him. How interesting that this God preferred honesty; in fact, the more real I was, the more real God was. Now that God was present and attentive, we could get down to the Work.

Looking within, I found that deep-down I desired to simply *be*. I knew that I would continue to act, but I wanted – needed – to eradicate the quid-pro-quo of working for money. I needed to act simply for the joy of it, and have my needs independently, unconditionally met, where money simply wasn't an issue.

"But, but..." came the objections. *"What about our Puritan work ethic? What about the fact that wealth does not always equal happiness?"* When my father had left NASA and General Electric's space program to start a small farm and antique shop in Maine, he was so much happier that our new poverty-level existence seemed infinitely blessed. And he had had a lot of scorn and contempt for those who remained in the rat-race at the expense of their souls. There were a lot of old programs to heal, including religious vows of poverty from what appeared to be past lives as well as my familial DNA.

But one by one, I integrated all the objections. *"It's OK,"* I told my wavicles. *"You can still have a Puritan work ethic, if you wish, and be independently wealthy. You can have infinite wealth and infinite happiness. You can have infinite wealth and a healthy and enlightened soul. You now take a powerful religious vow of prosperity. Your past lives and family DNA now*

9

completely support your independent wealth. You deserve to be supported for simply Being." And so on.

After two hours and many tears, I heard God say, "*Good! It is done; you have it!*" And I knew it was so, as my whole body hummed in contentment. I didn't know how it would manifest, but it was indeed done.

A few days later, my whole family unexpectedly received a trust fund that was supposed to have remained closed for several more generations. My share wasn't huge, but it was enough for room, board, and a little extra. My needs were met. My intellect quickly said, "Yeah, but surely that trust fund was going to open up anyway; it must have been on the way!" But as far as I can tell, it hadn't been. I had simply changed my reality to one where it *was* "on the way." Before the Wavicle Work on prosperity, I had needed to work for a living, and saw no way to change that. Afterwards, money was no longer an issue.

Ever since then, as other needs have arisen I have practiced some Wavicle Work, and Wholeness has always met those needs with infinite grace, usually through what appear afterward to be very natural means, but always in wonderful ways I couldn't have predicted or anticipated.

I have found that with Wavicle Work you have virtually no control over *how* the Work manifests into the physical plane. You are only responsible for giving the subtlest- and finest-feeling-level of accomplishment and perfection to your wavicles, and once they accept it, they will naturally manifest it in the most natural, life-supporting and holistic way.

Over the following 32 years I have repeatedly found myself practicing those same two forms of Wavicle Work: playing the part of Creator to our thought-creatures, and playing the part of creature to our Creator. Throughout all those years of helping myself and many others, Wavicle Work has remained the only technique I consistently use to create the desired reality. It is now my greatest pleasure to share it with you; I hope you will find it as wonderful a blessing as I do.

Chapter Two

The Art of Co-creation:
Wavicle Work in Seven Easy Steps

(1) *Realize that you are suffering – that something is not right in your creation.*

Acknowledge to yourself there is some need outside of you or inside of you which is not being met. Any thought of *I want...* or *I need...* actually comes from a wavicle, and is an opportunity to do some Wavicle Work to give yourself something important in order to grow, here and now. Be as honest as you can be with yourself. All your genuine needs are divinely planted, and in their fulfillment they bring about your further evolution and growth. The more truthful you are to yourself about your deepest need, the more quickly you can obtain it.

(2) *Take some deep, easy breaths and feel the emotional tension-point in your body associated with that need.*

Breathe, relax, and scan your body for the source of the need. This may move around in the body, as different sensations and emotions come to your attention, but in any given moment one point or area of tension will predominate. Simply place your attention on wherever the need is strongest in your body in any given moment. Trust the wisdom of your body in maintaining the perfect balance of what needs your attention most at this moment.

(3) *Imagine that the tension-point is itself doing the breathing.*

Put a nose on the tension-point and let it breathe in and out through your body in whatever manner it wishes: fast and shallow, slow and deep, or any other manner. Let it breathe the best, sweetest, most electrically life-filled air imaginable: golden,

11

sunny, redwood-scented mountain air, or an island-sunrise on-shore breeze, perhaps. This both establishes the tension-point as a separate entity and gives it loving support.

(4) *Imagine that tension-point as a separate little being or creature inside of you, a child of yours, and pay attention to it. Ask it what it needs.*

What does it look like? How does it feel? What does it most need in this moment? If you can't hear it clearly, you can ask it to speak louder, or show its feelings more strongly. If necessary, you can imagine that you shrink down and are that little being, communing with an all-loving form of your own higher self. Let this small I-particle be as honest and truthful as possible about how it feels and what it needs in this moment. Contrary to what you may have told it (or yourself) in the past, its needs ARE important: divine, God-given, God-planted, in fact, and they deserve to be met, here and now.

(5) *Relax again into your bigger Creator-self, your whole body-mind, and simply give that little being whatever it needs.*

You are bigger than it is; you contain it; you gave birth to it, and so for all intents and purposes you are its parent or its God. You are its immediate source of divine Love, divine Light, and divine Laughter. Your job is to play the part of the Creator, or divine parent, or Santa Claus, for that little being, giving it the experience of unconditional love, acceptance, and fulfillment. You can tell it:

"You are my divine child in whom my soul delights!

"Thank you so much for showing me these qualities of my Wholeness; I wouldn't be Whole without them. You have played your part absolutely perfectly.

"I am sorry I made you suffer so long; I am new to this God business. But I am here for you now and if you like, we can

12

change the past so that you remember it as but a story or a dream from which you have now awakened.

"I love you just as you are, unconditionally. I welcome you home to your perfect Heaven on Earth here and now, and I freely give you whatever you most need, now and forever. Your happiness is my happiness! What do you most need now?"

Whatever it needs, it's just a thought to you, and you can easily give it that thought, the fulfillment of that need. The perceived rules and limitations of three-dimensional Reality do not apply here. You are welcoming that wavicle back into its divine state and into its perfect paradise, however it may conceive that. It may be helpful to give it all the benefits of *opposites simultaneously*, as a way to fulfill its old programing completely while introducing a new one. For example, if a wavicle feels stuck in grief or constriction, you may say:

"If you wish it, I give you all the blessings and benefits of infinite grief and infinite joy simultaneously," or *"infinite constriction and infinite expansion simultaneously!"*

This brings your wavicle out of duality and into its Wholeness, which is *you*, the emptiful container of all possibilities.

(6) Imagine again that you are that little creature, breathing the fulfilment of your desire, and you are responding however you truly feel.

Relax, breathe, and scan your body. It will let you know how it is feeling and responding. However it feels, you simply allow that to be.

(7) If there is still some suffering or need, or some objection or "yeah-but" – and there probably will be – you simply repeat

the process, finding out who inside you needs what, and giving it to them.

Objections will naturally arise, as Wavicle Work changes your reality, your status quo, and so all the old programming still maintaining that status quo will present itself for healing or adjustment. It may well be helpful to ask your wavicles:

"Is there anyone here who objects to what we just gave that wavicle?"

Every objection your creature-wavicles offer you is an opportunity to refine and expand your gifts to them and hence to yourself. If you continue to identify with the objecting wavicles, your results will not be complete. The more of your objections you integrate, the more pure, real, and immediate your results are.

Playing the Part of the Creator

You don't need to feel the love, forgiveness, safety, rightness, etc., yourself before you give it to your wavicle. You may even think you are lying if you tell your wavicle these things, but you are not. You are actually telling a deeper truth than your intellect may be prepared to understand, and as your wavicle hears and recognizes that deeper truth your body begins to relax and feel more liberated: "The truth will set you free." Your wavicles connect you to your senses, and when they accept the truth, you too will feel that truth in your body, and from your body it will radiate out into your whole creation. So all you need to do is have the thought – the wavicle will receive the thought, accept it, and feel it, and then you will feel it through the wavicle.

The idea is to play the part of an unconditionally loving Creator for your creature-wavicles – not to simply replay the old programs of conditions, lack and limitation which your parents and society have given you. Those were doubtless absolutely perfect in their way, as they have created the perfect drama that you now enjoy, and now if you wish you can rewrite and improve on that perfection.

If you are not sure about playing the part of your own creator to your creature-particles, just take a leap of faith and do it. You can see yourself as an intermediary between your own infinitely loving God and your wavicles, if you prefer. That works equally well. But being your own original awareness, Wholeness, or God, is simply who you are, who you always have been, without your various layers of programming or beliefs. It is your original nondual *a priori* ground-state: very simple, easy, and natural. Whatever you are currently experiencing is simply how Wholeness looks and feels in this moment. It is both immanent and transcendental, conditioned and unconditional, "inside of" and "outside of" or unlimited by space and time, which means your simple awareness or Being or Wholeness has always been present, albeit perhaps for a time lost in identification with your more limited and separate personality.

Pretending to be Separate

It took a leap of faith, or at least an assumption, that you were separate from your infinite and eternal Wholeness to put a space-time program of separation in motion through eight successive steps or chakras of descent, precipitating from transcendence over your head (subtle spirit) down through your third-eye (middle spirit) and throat (dense spirit) into your heart (subtle soul), solar-plexus (middle soul) and navel (dense soul), and finally into your sex (subtle body), base (middle body), and feet (dense body). It will take an equal leap of faith or assumption to restore the original program and remember that after all, whatever you are experiencing in this moment, this too is Wholeness. This is simply how Wholeness or God happens to look and feel through your body-mind in this moment.

Experience may seem like a smooth unbroken flow of your separate I-ness inside a larger reality, but in actuality you are constantly — perhaps trillions of times a second — collapsing your

15

awareness from your Creator-field into your own creature-wavicles in order to experience the effects of your own thoughts through them, and to tangibly experience the creation you have created. This Creator-creature-creation dynamic will not be obvious if your awareness and conscious attention have been fixated solely in your creature-wavicles, lost in them and believing their programs and limitations to be your own, but nonetheless it is always happening.

A Whole New Movie

Each collapse into an I-wavicle is like a single movie-frame; your Creator-field is like the joins between the frames: normally invisible, but holding everything together. The frames run by swiftly enough, perhaps trillions per second, for you to ignore the joins and give yourself the illusion of a smooth movie. If you become aware of the joins, though, you can splice in different frames and create a whole new movie more to your conscious liking. If you want to experience or understand your own Creator-self, it is simply You, the neutral join between the movie-frames, the You behind your intellect and all of your beliefs.

To put it another way, you are the author and director of your movie, and your wavicles are like your actors. If you are done with your old movie, it may help to tell your suffering wavicle, **"Beautiful! That's a wrap! Now it is time for the cast party!"** The wavicle has indeed performed its part perfectly; it really had you believing in it! An amazing dream, but now it is time to awaken, if it chooses.

Your "Either-Or" Intellect is a Wavicle

Your intellect's function is to separate Wholeness – your own nature – into different choices and then make the "right" choice. This is absolutely necessary for creation; you would have no creation without duality, and your Wholeness desires to know

16

itself through your creation. Your intellect is a wonderful servant, but a painful master. It is itself a wavicle, a creature, a child or expression of Wholeness. When you identify with your intellect, you subject yourself to your intellect; losing touch with your Wholeness and identifying solely with a creature-wavicle, lost in duality-stories within your own Wholeness.

By believing your intellect and buying into the predominant duality of "good" and "bad," "better than" and "worse than," "I" and "not-I," "yesterday" and "tomorrow," you have eaten of the Tree of Knowledge of Good and Evil and thus expelled yourself from Paradise, identifying with a creature bound by space and time and hence mortal. Original sin is simply identification with spatial and temporal duality, and it occurs naturally when you as Wholeness lose Yourself in your own wavicle.

Identification with your own wavicle soon causes suffering, which is a wake-up call from your Wholeness to remember yourself, to awaken from your dream of separation. The whole time, You as Wholeness are always present, underlying Your own creation, all of it, both "good" and "bad." You may temporarily identify with the creature-you who rejoices in the "good" and suffers in the "bad," but the Creator-You is never truly lost. You can consciously regain and realize your ever-present underlying Wholeness and perfect Paradise, your Kingdom of Heaven within you, your own eternal Life of infinite abundance, by doing Wavicle Work.

Erasing Karma with Grace by Wavicle Work

Karma is a great story. From the point of view of a wavicle, Karma – the law of action and reaction in space-time – certainly exists. *But karma is only a refusal to love Here and Now.* Let go of your wavicle's belief in space-time and you can be in any world you want, as you contain all worlds, all possibilities. From the point of view of Wholeness, there is only Here and Now, which you automatically extend both into the past as a supporting story, and into the future as anticipated results. With

17

Wavicle Work you can jump from one reality to another, from one timeline to another. When you choose your new timeline, you automatically create or "discover" a whole new history to support it.

Life is like a dream. Your dreaming mind is capable of constructing an entire back-story in a microsecond, as when you are experiencing a lengthy dream which along the way may establish a seemingly logical and rational cause for an external stimulus. For example, you dream you have obtained a wonderful new job across the country and so you are now moving out of your old apartment, and after loading all of your furniture into your rented moving-van and driving it to your new house, which looks amazing, you are now taking the truck up your driveway in reverse, making a *beep-beep-beep* sound which as you awaken you realize is your alarm clock. It is as if your mind heard the sound and instantly provided a whole history to precede and explain it. Karma is like that.

By loving your wavicles, you erase karma, breathing grace from the infinite realm of all possibilities and all stories, into the finite arena of space-time to create or recreate and enjoy a specific story.

Wavicle Work supersedes the Law of Karma with the Law of Grace.

Chapter Three

Particle Prayer

Sometimes you may feel too overwhelmed to do Wavicle Work from the point of view of the Creator, or you may simply want to experience the relationship more fully from the other side. If so, you may focus on Chapter Two's Step Four, and practice *Particle Prayer*: play the part of the particle, the creature, and imagine your Creator is not you.

For this relationship to work, you will have to allow a God that is larger than the impersonal Absolute – large enough in fact to care personally about you: large enough for that Wholeness to "collapse" into an omniscient, omnipresent, omnipotent I AM, to assume a personality, to bend a compassionate and loving interest toward each one of the tiny creatures in creation, including you.

If you prefer, you don't have to *believe* in such a God; simply *imagine* it. That will do the job. Imagine your God as occupying a tangible form, with a tangible presence. If you allow your God to be truly omnipotent, he or she or they will be able to manifest through matter as easily as through spirit. Here are the steps to perform Particle Prayer:

(A) *Realize you are suffering.*

Let go of your defenses and your denials, take some deep breaths, relax, and let yourself admit you are in pain, or that there is something you need in this moment.

(B) *Establish a safe space to open and earth yourself.*

There are many ways to approach prayer. You may have your own favorites. I sometimes like to prepare to connect with the Wholeness or Holiness of God with the "Triple Sun Technique." Imagine the Central Spiritual Sun of the Universal Father as a radiantly golden source of Love a few feet over your head, and the Central Material Sun of the Earth Mother or Mother Nature as another radiantly golden source of Love a few feet below your feet.

Now feel both of these Suns pouring warm golden flows of love and light into you from above and below, healing everything in their path and meeting in your Sacred Heart (your Solar Plexus, midway between your heart and navel), where they ignite the "I AM" of your Inner Central Sun, which then radiates brilliantly and ecstatically out in all directions to illuminate and heal your entire world and everyone in it. If you like, you can time the inpouring with your in-breath, and the out-flooding with your out-breath.

This technique both opens you to divine Spirit and earths you to divine Matter, so you remain balanced and grounded, able to handle divine energies running through your body and into your creation without the risk of overload or burnout. If practicality permits, practicing the technique with your bare feet on the ground or in the ocean enhances your physical grounding immensely.

Here are a few experiences from students practicing the Triple Sun Technique:

"Sitting in the middle of the room ... I could feel the energy pouring through me, which was pretty fantastic, and my heart expanded a lot, which is a rare experience for me, and it was obviously ... pretty joyful...." — C. T.

"What I just experienced ... was an immense amount of light. It was just so present ... there was nothing fake about it. When I felt the energies combining it really felt like a burst of light outside of my eyes and I wanted to open my eyes just to see if someone was shining a flashlight on me or something — I didn't, but that's what it felt like. It was really powerful.... I felt this "pushing out" and I felt almost like this manifestation of laughter just flowing out. Really good. I never felt anything like that. Thank you for facilitating it." — S. L.

"I invoked the Center of Divine Love perched atop the subtle chakra system extending from the crown, asking that center to infuse me with its Love. I then felt that energy trickling down into my solar plexus, after which time the energy merged with the same energy ascending up the lower chakras from the center of the earth. Once the two energy streams met, though, there was an explosion of light and high-frequency sound which then immediately circulated around the circumference of an expanding energy disk existing perpendicularly to my body. As the meditation continued, strong currents of bliss ran through my brow and crown chakras. The brain felt like it was being illuminated with invisible light. I then experienced that everything in my environment—all the sounds, objects, people—became part of my own awareness, suffusing everything with the most intimate and tender Love.

"Then, I [opened my eyes] just to corroborate this experience. To my wonder the entire environment was submerged in a three-foot-high energy field of gentle bluish-white light, from which everything and everyone emerged, but without ever losing their status as nodes of the Unmanifest. My very own Awareness. All moved in slow motion, it seemed, in distinct frames, as if every nanosecond of manifestation were being brought into being, maintained, and then dissolved. The entire spectacle was Love on the move. I was That. The universe was inside me: the Heart of the cosmos. What a big 'Wow!' all of this was.

"Since that time, the experience has returned at different levels of intensity." — M. B.

(C) *Open to Your Creator's unconditional Love.*

Now let's open to the infinite Love of your Creator. You can imagine your Creator listening to you unconditionally, pouring love down like olive-oil or honey into your mind and heart, or surging up from the earth in waves of nourishing love, or loving you in the form of your own fully-grown self a million years from now. Eventually, in all eternity, you will solve any given issue or problem; go to your future self where the desired outcome has already happened, and download that subtle information or finest-feeling-level into the present.

You can say, *"I open myself to the highest* (or *deepest,* or *truest*) *vibration* (or *reality*) *that is comfortable for me in this moment."* Then relax, breathe, and feel the results. *Don't* forget the *"that is comfortable"* part; it is very important.

You can use statements like, "I open myself to my Creator," and "I and my Creator are One," and "I AM my Creator," to begin to strengthen the connection between your creature-self and your Creator-self.

Remember, this is not an earthly parent you are imagining with the typical earthly "ought" and "should" programs of conditioning, criticism, and limitation; this is your Creator, your Wholeness, your larger self: all-loving, all-knowing and all-blissful, and loving and knowing and delighting in you unconditionally, exactly as you are. If you find yourself imagining a Deity who doesn't care about you, or is judgmental, feel free to respectfully "discharge" Him or Her, with thanks for past service, and connect with One who is large enough to be able to care about and truly love the relatively small things in Life, like you in your creature-self, just as you are.

Your God may be either above or below you, behind or before you, to the left or the right of you, around you or within you, or all of the above. Regardless of where you might imagine your Creator to be, simply imagine or sense a golden love-flow of current between you and your Creator.

If you are having difficulties sensing your Creator, simply ask yourself, *"If* my unconditionally loving Creator were here now, paying attention to me, what would it feel like?" This is a good way to bypass your internal censor whose job it is to preserve the status quo. It doesn't mind allowing alternate realities for you as long as you reassure it they are only what-ifs.

You can also use the Creator's wonderful multiplicity of creatures to amplify your experience. Consciously breathe in sunlight and moonlight and starlight to heal and nourish you: any or all of them, day or night; they are all always present and available to you.

Open to the divine life and loving energy in subtle earth and food. Open to the subtle water of life surging up, or sprinkling or pouring down onto and into you. Open to the loving vitality of the subtle air around and within you. Open to the purifying ecstasy of the subtle sun-like fire in every atom, or step into a loving column of immortal fire. All are happy to help you if you open to them.

Crystals, metals, herbs, trees, animals, and birds can all be very useful; simply treat them as you would like to be treated: as if they are conscious, loving, intelligent beings, and ask them to help you. Masters, Ancestors, Angels, Elementals, Saints, and Gods and Goddesses of love, light, and laughter are always ready on the subtle planes to help you as well, if you ask. Every one of them is a wavicle of your Wholeness, waiting to be of service to you. Every being, every wavicle in your Creation, is an aspect of your Creator, an aspect of your own Self.

Exercise discrimination and respect your own boundaries: if you encounter energies or personalities that are not completely to your liking and you don't wish to accept or integrate them right now, feel free to respectfully refuse them, and ask for and open to ones that feel more unconditionally loving, enlightened, and joyous, or simply more comfortable for you. While at some point you as Wholeness will probably "digest" every energy and integrate it back into love, you are not required to do it all right now. Ask your Wholeness to take care of it for you. Space and time are also here to serve you; you contain them, and you have all of infinity and eternity in which to accomplish and achieve everything you desire.

(D) *In Love, tell your truth.*

When you feel you have established a connection with your Creator, in loving honesty tell your Creator how you truly feel and what you truly need, being as truthful as you can be about your deepest desires. It can be painful to resurrect desires you have deeply buried and tried to ignore as being too impractical or immoral. *But the more real you are as a creature, the more real your Creator will be.* As it says in the Yoga Sutras, *"When Truth is established, all acts will achieve their desired results."*

If you feel sad or confused, tell your Creator that. If you feel guilty or frustrated or angry, tell your Creator that. Remember, in playing the part of a creature, *you are a wave of your Creator's Ocean of Love. Love is the carrier-wave of Truth. Truth sets you free.*

(E) *Open to your Creator's loving message for you.*

Breathe, relax, and feel how your body responds to the unconditional love of your Creator. Again, if you are having difficulty doing so, you can simply ask yourself, *"If* my Creator were unconditionally loving me right now, how would it feel, and what would my Creator be telling me?" This will generally bypass your internal censor, who is attempting to maintain your status-quo reality for you.

(F) *Keep communicating until your body, mind, and spirit are satisfied.*

Continue with the process of breathing, attuning, and communing until you feel satisfied and complete on every level: physically vital, emotionally content, mentally clear, intuitively centered, and spiritually inspired. Various forms of yoga, including meditation and selfless service, may speed your progress and deepen your results. Follow your intuition, your awakened heart.

"Be Ye Perfect, Even as Your Father in Heaven is Perfect"

Your needs are God-given; they are divine seeds-of-growth, and despite your programming to the contrary (also perfect in its way), you as a creature are made perfect, in God's image, as the well-deserving and well-loved child of God, in whom God is well pleased. You have always done the best you could do in any given moment, and thus you are always doing God's will – which has been, in fact, perfect in its own way. Even your mistakes and suffering are perfect in that they serve to teach you and awaken you from full identification with your dream.

It is not fair to you to second-guess yourself after the fact and punish yourself for not doing at the time what appeared later to be the right choice. At any given moment, you are doing your very best, given your often-conflicting desires, and that is providing experience for Wholeness, Reality, or God. And that is all that Wholeness really asks of you as a creature – that you be a sense-organ, an individuated experiencer, an angel or a devata, of Wholeness for Wholeness.

So you may choose to identify primarily either with creature or with Creator in doing Wavicle Work; it works either way if you are honest about your needs and imagine a strong connection between both Creator and creature. When that Creator-creature flow is present, miracles happen.

When Not to Do Wavicle Work

In general, it is good to do Wavicle Work whenever a suffering wavicle comes to your attention. With practice, you can do a little Wavicle Work whenever the opportunity presents itself, even in activity if you have a few moments. It's not a good idea to divide your attention if you are out in the world doing something that requires concentration, but often the simplest form of WW, *"I love you, I love you, I love you; you're mine, you're mine, you're mine!"* or even just an imagined hug of a suffering wavicle will suffice. Not merely positive thinking, your love actually appears to reprogram your body's cells and DNA back into coherently harmonious and healthy light-wavicles, resolving the suffering into bliss. At least, that's how it looks to me.

There may well be times when you are too caught up in the internal drama to remember to do either form of Wavicle Work. That's OK; it is only possible to do WW when you can remember to do it. When you have sufficient clarity and remember, and you actually have a choice whether to practice it or not, then you can do WW, if you wish. It can be best to practice WW in a quiet time and place, like a meditation or prayer.

Of course, you don't need to do Wavicle Work if you are enjoying the particular drama you have created. Life is like a dream, or a movie: if you are enjoying it, you don't need to keep repeating, "It's only a movie!" It's only when you are suffering in a nightmare that you might wish to wake up, withdraw the senses into the body, feel the tension-point "in here" associated with the issue "out there," and give the wavicle what it most needs, thus changing the movie.

Wavicle Work is not intended as a substitute for any traditional methods of healing or advice, including medical, psychotherapeutic, or economic: I recommend you always consult and follow the advice of your preferred professional specialists as it resonates with your truth; they are a part of your Wholeness and here to help you.

And of course, most importantly, Wavicle Work is for internal use only. The freedom you accord your wavicles in your inner world is not to be expressed as license in your outer world, where regular social strictures and laws apply. Such an application would be ineffectual and counter-productive.

Chapter Four

Using Wavicle Work for Passion, Prosperity, Dharma, and Liberation

Depending on the "elements" in their constitution, wavicles may come to your attention with any of four primary goals: Fiery wavicles are here to ignite Passion, the blessings of intense desire. Earthy wavicles embody to seek and acquire Prosperity, the blessings of wealth and abundance. Airy wavicles are present to balance Dharma, the blessings of right action and justice. Watery wavicles are here to surrender into Liberation, the blessings of dissolving all limitations into freedom.

People often have mixed constitutions and identify with more than one of these goals, either all at once or over time, and it is certain that Wavicle Work will eventually uncover wavicles or devatas in you desiring all of them.

Sometimes people believe that if they achieve only one of these goals, they will automatically obtain all of them: Follow your passion and you will find freedom, for example, or find your dharma and you will automatically obtain prosperity. Such is not the case. Passion may free you from some strictures, but by itself can actually imprison or enslave you. And almost everyone knows a born care-giver who has a hard time accepting gifts in return. They are in their dharma and quite comfortable giving, but not as comfortable with receiving wealth.

Also, each of the four primary goals has three possible qualifiers: Love, Light, and Laughter. Thus your wavicle may more specifically desire Loving, Enlightened, or Blissful Passion, Wealth, Dharma, or Liberation. Asking your wavicles what they most need is paramount, and they usually need something quite specific, but occasionally you might run all of twelve of these possibilities by your wavicles and see if any really lights them up or evokes a *Yes!*

27

For best results in Wavicle Work and a well-balanced life, be alert and responsive to whatever your wavicles need whenever your wavicles present them. Feeling the accomplishment of these goals internally on every level naturally prepares you to accept them gracefully in a life-supporting way when they materialize externally.

Passion

As the Wholeness from which your wavicles emerged and into which they long to return, you are their ultimate passion and chief desire. All true desires are evolutionary, and meeting your wavicles' immediate desires on the subtle, inner, finest-feeling level helps them quickly regain their ultimate passion for and enjoyment of harmony and unity with you.

Passion has acquired a bad reputation in spiritual circles that advocate the cessation of all desire. Self-described *advaitins* or nondualists may tell you that they ignore their thoughts and desires as "just a story." But if you are truly nondual, you will realize that your thoughts and desires are your wavicles and just as much a part of Wholeness as everything else. All of creation is "just a story," including the belief that you are beyond all that. Ignorance of your wavicles is a form of resistance, and whatever you resist, persists. If you ignore or try to suppress a suffering wavicle, it will continue to nag you.

Yes, a part of you is an eternal, unchanging, Absolute no-self in Nirvana. But a part of you is a temporary, ever-changing, Relative self in suffering or Samsara. Favoring one over the other is dualism. True nondualism reveals that this apparent duality is itself just a story; the Absolute and Relative need each other to co-exist, and ultimately Nirvana is Samsara; Samsara is Nirvana. Spirit and Matter are one. Wavicle Work is all about separating yourself from your wavicle to get an overview of it, in order to love it unconditionally and bring it into harmony and unity with you. That includes honoring and fulfilling all of your wavicle's deepest desires, no matter how arcane. Remember,

28

Wavicle Work is all done internally, so you can give your wavicles anything. If you are truly fulfilling their deepest needs, only love and harmony will manifest into your material creation.

In truth your desires are just as important as anything (or Nothing) else. Desires and their fulfilment are crucial for your wavicles to enjoy the benefits of space-time and evolution. Again, you are the deepest desire of your wavicles, as you are their Wholeness, their source and ultimate goal, but they may not come to you if you don't love them where they are. Withholding your love from them "freezes" them until you do love them right where they are, as your perfect creation.

Wavicle Work points out that the problem is not your desire, it is your whole-hearted identification with it and/or your outright rejection of it that causes you suffering. That is because when you either identify with or reject your desire, you are taking the dualistic point of view of a specific wavicle: one small creature in a large and alien universe. This is not the whole truth, and so Grace nudges you to awaken and remember your Wholeness.

If you ignore the first mental nudges to awaken, and persist in thinking yourself only a wavicle, Grace will give you stronger nudges, which may feel like emotional distress. If you ignore those too and continue your story, Grace will give you still stronger nudges, which may appear as physical unease or disease. If you are deeply asleep in the wavicle, you may interpret those friendly nudges as an attack, and feel suffering.

For best results, when you are nudged, start doing Wavicle Work; give your wavicles your unconditional loving attention; welcome them home to Heaven on Earth, and let them know you are fulfilling all of their deepest desires here and now. And by immediately fulfilling those desires internally on the subtlest and finest feeling level, you are erasing karma. Grace resulting from completed Wavicle Work is automatic and life-supporting, and flows from the pre-existent Wholeness and fullness you have established, not from an empty or addictive craving or mental attempts to control external events.

Passion is often tied to Prosperity or Abundance; many wavicles feel they cannot follow or obtain their true Passion without infinite Prosperity. You can remind them that you are here to fulfill all of their desires easily and effortlessly, here and now, including their desires for abundance. Let's take a closer look at Prosperity:

Prosperity

Prosperity is abundance of all kinds, not merely wealth: family, friends, and health are generally your most important forms of prosperity. As your wavicles' Creator and parent, potential best friend, and ultimate Wholeness, you are truly their prosperity. As their programmer on the finest-feeling level, you are also their ultimate source of more tangible wealth. It is you who gives or withholds permission for them to allow wealth into their and your life.

Like passion, prosperity has also acquired a bad reputation among spiritual seekers who see an unbridgeable gulf between Spirit above and Matter below, with the Soul in the middle having to choose between them. "Money is the root of all evil," they may say, which is actually a misquote of "The *love* of money is the root of all evil." If you love anything more than God or your own Wholeness, or as separate from Wholeness, then you have given that thing (or its lack) the power to overshadow your Wholeness, to overshadow your *good*. But from Wholeness's point of view, in truth, there is only good; Spirit and Matter are One; Wholeness alone *is*.

Another puzzling Biblical saying is, "Blessed are the poor in spirit, for theirs is the kingdom of Heaven." You could say this means those wavicles are blessed who humbly know they are in need and are open to receive divine abundance from Wholeness, for they shall receive the riches of Heaven, on the finest-feeling level, here and now. As their emptiful Wholeness, *you* are their divine abundance, their kingdom of Heaven. From their point of view you are Brahman, the Nothing and Everything, and so *you*

30

are truly the poor in spirit, the one who does not even own a separate self, or wholly identify with your wavicles.

The desire for abundance is legitimate, and it deserves to be fulfilled here and now, in your Heaven on Earth. Money is absolutely neutral, like electricity, which can either electrocute you or keep your house comfortable. Wavicle Work that properly integrates all of your devatas' objections immediately fulfills their divine desire to experience wealth, giving them the subtle, finest-feeling level of infinite abundance. In this utter contentment and integrity there is no desire to steal, and as the Yoga Sutras say, *"When Non-stealing* (or *"integrity"*) *is established, all riches flow."*

At first glance, this saying about abundance in the Bible might seem very unfair: *"For whoever has, to him shall be given, and he shall have more abundance: but whoever has not, from him shall be taken away even what he has."* But on the subtlest-feeling level it makes perfect sense: If you put your attention on what you have and on the finest-feeling level of infinite abundance in all gratitude, you are instructing your wavicles to manifest more abundance. If you put your attention on what you don't have and on the finest-feeling level of lack, you are instructing your wavicles to manifest more poverty.

Here is a friend's experience after one Wavicle Work session on prosperity:

"I recently enjoyed my first one-on-one session [and] we worked on addressing the needs of and loving my wealth and prosperity wavicles. I was empowered and relieved of my past fears of never being able to spend money freely and always feeling a lack of money even when I have had savings in the bank. The week following my personal session I began noticing that I was more relaxed and able to spend money more freely. I was even able to feel good about giving gifts to myself and to others... actions [that] would have been very difficult and would have caused me a lot of mental discomfort and anxiety.

"But the real surprise came just a few days later. A letter came in the mail saying that there was a program I might be eligible for to receive an extra $100 a month, and that I should fill out a bunch of paperwork and send it in. However, before I even took any action, the next day I received a new letter that stated I was automatically enrolled in the program; the money would automatically show up in my account, and that there was nothing additional that I needed to do. This brought me great internal joy, but that was just the beginning of an amazing transformation that soon began to reveal itself in my 'external world' as well.

"A few days after I received the second letter ... I was delightfully surprised to learn that a family trust had opened up and my family would now be receiving an ongoing stipend worth over $60,000. On learning this news, I laughed and laughed with pure delight because I know full well that my wealth wavicle was truly feeling loved and appreciated in new ways and was now beginning and continuing to infinitely orchestrate spontaneous wealth for me. In just a matter of a very few days my entire relationship to money and prosperity had gotten substantially better. And due to Rory's healing technology I now enjoy an enriched spirit-mind-body in so many practical ways. Thanks ... for teaching me how to heal my inner and outer Self. With sincere appreciation."– R. O.

Prosperity is often closely tied to Dharma, or right-action; many wavicles don't believe that they deserve wealth because they have done wrong, or that they would misuse wealth if they obtained it. You may wish to assure your wavicles that they have always done right and will always automatically use their infinite abundance for the highest good of all. Let's look at Dharma more closely:

Dharma

Dharma is right action, behaving in accord with natural law, the law of Wholeness. You are the Wholeness of your wavicles; your thoughts are their law, and your wavicles naturally desire to behave in accord with your law or your will. However, as you have consciously or unconsciously rejected and hurt many of them, they feel they must have done something terribly wrong, although in truth they have always done exactly what you consciously or unconsciously asked them to do.

It is up to you as their Creator to apologize for hurting them and to reassure them that they have always done exactly as you have asked; that they have always done their very best in any given moment; that their best has always been utterly perfect, as they have always brought you more experiences and expanded your knowledge, which is all you have asked of them.

Those who have "died" or had near-death experiences, have seen their life from a radical, new perspective and come back to Earth inevitably appreciating that true dharma is not so much grandiose plans and earth-shaking deeds as it is the countless little things you do moment-to-moment: the dollar you give a homeless man, the smile you give a stranger, the unconditional love you naturally emanate. But this constant grace flows most naturally from the inner fullness of a strong Creator-creature flow, such as you give and receive in Wavicle Work. The desire to express your gifts in your perfect dharma is natural and God-given, and one that your wavicles naturally deserve from you.

You may have no idea how your dharma is going to manifest; simply give your wavicles exactly what they need, here and now, on the inner, finest-feeling level. A friend of mine who is a master of Eurythmy, Rudolf Steiner's expressive movement art, very specifically desired a group of six trained eurythmists with whom to do research and practice Eurythmy, even though she was living in a town and state that knew next to nothing of Steiner or his Waldorf Schools. To her this request seemed impossible.

She did Wavicle Work on her dharma, gave her wavicles what they needed, and within a few days received a call out of the blue from a Waldorf School in another state, inviting her to come and teach Eurythmy. Besides the full-time teaching position with benefits, as an added bonus there were six eurythmists in the area who invited her to work with them in a weekly exploration into deeper aspects of Eurythmy including artistic work.

When asked how the Waldorf School had come to call her, she replied, "You know, I never asked them. The woman who contacted me didn't tell me. But Eurythmy/Waldorf is a small world and probably someone recommended she call. I had told some people that I felt underutilized. I had put an ad in Waldorf Jobs, but they don't give out phone numbers ... so, I am not really sure."

This is an excellent example of how Wavicle Work often manifests: beforehand your goal seems utterly impossible, but after you have changed timelines, your new reality may come with a backstory making your miracle seem completely natural if not inevitable.

Dharma is often closely tied to Liberation; many wavicles feel that right action would be constraining, so it is good to let them know that right action is easy, effortless, automatic, comfortable, and liberating. Now let's take a closer look at Liberation:

Liberation

Liberation is transcendence, freedom, the process of escaping the bonds of a prior program or belief-structure and its resultant reality. As you are the infinite Wholeness of your wavicles, you are their ultimate liberation. Just as your old programs and their limitations were merely a thought, so is liberation: easily given to your wavicles, but with potentially radical and fundamental paradigm-shifting results.

Many times a wavicle will actually fear liberation, as it believes the new reality will not be as simple, easy, safe, comfortable, fun, or popular as the status quo. If so, you can readily assure your wavicle that its new liberation will be even simpler, easier, safer, more comfortable, more fun, and more popular than ever before. You can let your wavicle know that if it wishes, it can enjoy all the blessings and benefits of the current program of limitation together with unconditional and infinite liberation, simultaneously, now and forever.

A friend dedicated one session of Wavicle Work to liberating herself from an addiction to caffeine. After giving her wavicles what they really needed and wished to get from coffee, she reported that she effortlessly quit that same day, and to her surprise remained happily caffeine-free for months afterward. She also reported that while she had depended upon coffee to give her the energy she needed to get all of her work done, now she still accomplished all of her daily tasks, and in a much smoother and easier way than she ever had done with coffee. She also found that her smiles were brighter and more sincere, and that people had started asking her what she was doing differently.

Occasionally a dedicated practitioner of Wavicle Work will suddenly experience an unexpected purposelessness or absence of desire, as if everything has just revealed itself to be essentially, absolutely, and always the same unchanging reality. This sameness is a natural result of a wavicle's complete liberation from its old program, belief, or drama. It is the wavicle's first taste of the infinity of possibilities simultaneously inherent in Wholeness, and is generally followed by a permanent and infinitely deep relief, freedom, contentment, and enjoyment along with subsequently even more effective wavicle-work and manifestation.

Liberation is often closely tied to Passion; many wavicles fear that Liberation will be passionless or that they will be required to sacrifice their desires to obtain Liberation. You can reassure them that liberation is fluid, always allowing for more and more growth and perfection, and creating ever easier and swifter fulfilment of all of their desires throughout all of eternity. With that in mind, you may wish to revisit the section on Passion, at the beginning of this chapter. Or you may wish to go on to the next chapter, which will suggest some ways to heal some of the more commonly-encountered demons or suffering wavicles back into their truer nature as your happy, healthy angels.

Chapter Five

Converting Your Demons into Angels

A wavicle may appear to be within you in the form of an emotion, thought, or belief, or outside of you in the form of a person, animal, corporation, political party, or the like. Either way, no matter what it looks like, it is simply an emanation of your consciousness, and you can treat all troublesome or suffering wavicles the same way: withdraw the senses from "out there" to the associated pain or tension-point "in here" in the body, let the tension-point breathe, and then treat it as your beloved child, your angel, your devotee or devata.

Every demon is simply an angel to whom you have given a dirty job: to show you some quality of yourself, of your Wholeness, that you don't yet understand and probably don't like. Like everything, they respond very well to unconditional love, and when you give them the opportunity they quickly and joyously become your devatas or devotees again. In fact they always have been; you just forgot what you asked them to do.

Can you imagine how odd it must be for them? You asked them to perform a specific unpleasant task, and when they play the part perfectly, you reject them for performing it so well! It's as if you had cast Anthony Hopkins to play Hannibal Lector in *Silence of the Lambs* and forever after you have shunned the Oscar-winning actor as a psychopathic cannibal.

Here are some of the more common demons and some ways to integrate them and convert them back into angels.

Anger and Wavicle Work

Anger and ulcers are the shadow-side or underside of zeal, "fire in the belly," loving passion, strength, animal spirits, clairvoyance, and a sense of divine timing: all gifts you may be refusing yourself if you refuse to love anger unconditionally as an integral part of your Wholeness and Holiness.

Impatience, irritability, resentment, anger, and rage are signs that a wavicle's deepest needs have not been met. You have probably been running "sensible" programs applying learned three-dimensional limitations to a being who is a quantum wavicle: essentially a devata, an angel or a divine emanation, a child of Wholeness or God.

You may have been telling your wavicle that it shouldn't have those deep needs, or that you cannot fulfill them. But the wavicle's needs are divine needs, and deserve to be treated with the utmost respect, and to be fulfilled here and now. On the interior, finest-feeling level, which is abstract to you but utterly tangible to your wavicle, you can always give it exactly what it most needs, *now*.

If your creature-wavicle feels impatient, angry, or enraged you can tell it:

"Thank you for bringing this to my attention! I honor your impatience, anger, and rage; these feelings are a part of our Wholeness; I wouldn't be Whole without them, and I love you whole-heartedly and welcome you home just as you are to your perfect Heaven on Earth. I want you to know I am here for you to meet your needs fully and unconditionally, here, now, and always. What do you most need?"

If a wavicle feels destructive, you can tell it:

"Many thanks for showing me this desire to destroy; it is a part of my Wholeness and I wouldn't be whole without it! Your need to destroy is necessary, and I honor and love you whole-heartedly and unconditionally just as you are. I need destruction to enjoy creation. I need destruction to enjoy purification. I need destruction to enjoy a perfect immune system. Thank you for doing such a great job! If you like, I give you

all the benefits and blessings of infinite destruction and infinite creation simultaneously, or an entire world for you to destroy to your heart's content, or whatever else you most need. Welcome home! What do you most need?"

If you feel it is appropriate, don't hesitate to give your wavicles a separate inner world, a bubble or "play-pen" in your awareness-field to act out their desires to their heart's content. Separation is a part of your Wholeness. And just as the three-dimensional rules of the outer world don't apply to the inner one, you don't translate the freedoms of the inner world into licentious acts in the outer one.

Greed, Craving, Addiction, and Wavicle Work

Greed is the shadow-side of receptivity, groundedness in heart-felt faithful gratitude, and radiantly enlightened prosperity, all gifts you may be refusing to receive if you refuse to accept greed as an integral part of your Wholeness.

If the wavicle feels greedy, or is afraid you will spoil it if you give it all it needs, simply tell it:

"Your greed is a part of my Wholeness, and I wouldn't be complete without it! Thank you so much for showing it to so beautifully! One is only spoiled when one gets what one doesn't really need instead of what one does. I adore you; I love you just as you are! I now give you, freely and unconditionally, exactly what you most need, on every level including the tangible level of the senses, here and now and always! You are my divine child, and I welcome you home to your perfect Heaven on Earth. What do you most need?"

You may also tell your wavicle:

"It is easy, safe, and comfortable for you to receive everything you most need, now and forever. Thank you so much for being you! Welcome home, to your perfect Heaven on Earth, now and forever! What do you most need in this moment?"

What you are ultimately craving is not really a particular experience or object; it is simply perfect Love, the merger of your Self "in here" with your Self "out there" – which is only realized through comprehending the equal perfection of both "in here" and "out there." Your sacred heart will connect you, but it has ultimate integrity; it will not unite you with anything you are telling yourself is less than perfect. But that idea of imperfection is simply a story you superimposed over a portion of the perfect Wholeness you already are, and everything already *is*.

An addiction is a program which says you have to do something physical or get something concrete "out there" in order to obtain the subtle feeling you most desire "in here." Often a wavicle perceives its (and your) Wholeness as only *empty*, not *emptiful*, and then fruitlessly tries to "avoid the Void" and fill it with an addiction. The truth is, you can always give your creatures whatever subtle feeling they need "in here" right now, and then whatever action may still be required "out there" will flow naturally out of fullness and contentment rather than emptiness and craving.

As Jesus says, "Seek ye first the kingdom of God and his righteousness [i.e., Wholeness and its perfection], and all else will be added unto you." Wholeness is always available within, unconditionally, on the finest-feeling level of your heart. Krishna similarly says, "Established in Union with the divine (or Wholeness), perform action."

Addictions are disempowering, as you are making your own inner satisfaction contingent upon some external event. Again, an addictive wavicle is trying to *do* something or *get* something "out there" in order to *feel* something "in here." Sometimes the wavicles fear that they won't accomplish anything "out there" unless they are suffering "in here". But really they suffer only to get your attention; once you give your wavicles their fulfilment "in here," action continues automatically to reflect your inner state of contentment "out there." If you find yourself acting in an addictive way, simply bless and love whatever you are doing, and offer your wavicle immediate fulfillment of its deepest desires, unconditionally, inwardly, here and now.

You can tell your wavicle:

"Your addiction is a part of my Wholeness, and I wouldn't be Whole without it. Thank you so much for showing it to me so beautifully; you really had me believing in it! I love you unconditionally; you are my divine child in whom my soul delights, and I am here now to welcome you home to Heaven on Earth and to give you what you most need, unconditionally, now and forever!"

What does your wavicle *really* need? The addiction is only a *metaphor* for its true satisfaction. Go beyond the symbolic act; go deeper and ask and give your wavicle what it most truly needs, here and now.

In a way, you are like a spirit-guide, and your suffering wavicles are like lost souls, people who have died and are not clear on what happens next. They are like addicts, like ghosts, in that they are still attached to the physical world because of an unmet desire. Your job is to let these souls know they are in good hands, and they now can have all their addictive desires met, and come into the Light – which is your unconditionally loving attention – and come Home, to whatever paradise they most desire.

You can even use a traditional prayer for healing such ghosts, slightly adapted for wavicle work:

"Dearly beloved friend, you are healed and forgiven; you are one with your own higher nature; you are one with your own greatest self; you are one with me. I have come to take you to

41

your perfect place, your own perfect heaven of love, light and laughter now. Come in peace, and welcome home."

Lying, Denigration, and Wavicle Work

Lying, "bad-mouthing," cursing (in the sense of disparaging or blighting), and denigration are the shadow-side of truth-telling, authenticity, magic, throat-laughter, poetry, and blissfully ecstatic right-action and hopeful justice – all gifts you may be refusing yourself if you refuse to love lying and denigration unconditionally as an integral part of your Wholeness and Holiness.

If a wavicle is a liar, or is bad-mouthing someone or something, you can tell it:

"Your lying and bad-mouthing are a part of my Wholeness, and I wouldn't be Whole without them! Thank you so much for showing me these parts of myself. You have done a magnificent job! You are a wonderful actor. I love you unconditionally, just as you are! You may continue this role for as long as you like, or you may set it aside as the dream it is and rest in the blissful expression of your own deepest truth and power. You are my devata, you are divine, your speech is magical, and your universe and all of its inhabitants are full of true love and holiness and divinity! Welcome home to Heaven on Earth!"

.

Unpopularity, Insanity, and Wavicle Work

Unpopularity, insanity, and "water on the brain" are the shadow-sides of loving temperance and liberation, bodily containment of the Whole of creation, and a "fluid mind," an awareness of and sensitivity to the very subtlest lunar wisdom: all of which

42

you may be denying yourself if you refuse to allow unpopularity and insanity to be legitimate parts of your Wholeness.

If you encounter a wavicle who feels unpopular or insane you may tell it:

"Your unpopularity and insanity are a part of my Wholeness, and I wouldn't be whole without them! Many thanks for showing them to me so clearly. You are my beloved child in whom my soul delights, and I love you unconditionally. If you like, you may maintain these roles forever, or you may gently and comfortably awaken from them now into the deeper truth of infinite love and appreciation and respect, for you are divine, and have always been divinely popular and perfectly healthy just as you are, and everyone in your world loves you deeply and acknowledges your perfect Wholeness. Welcome home to your perfect Heaven on Earth, now and forever!"

Pride, Solipsism, and Wavicle Work

Pride, arrogance, "hot-headedness," and solipsism are the shadow-sides of faithful self-sufficiency, the "fire in the head" of creative solar imagination, and radiantly enlightened passion: all gifts you may be refusing yourself if you refuse to allow pride and solipsism a place in your Wholeness.

If you encounter a proud or solipsistic wavicle you may tell it:

"Your pride and solipsism are a part of my Wholeness, and I wouldn't be Whole without them! Thank you so much for showing me these flavors of myself. You are my devata in whom my soul delights! I love you unconditionally, just as you are, and am here to give you whatever you most need, now and forever. If you wish you may keep these flavors of pride and solipsism forever, or you may enjoy all the benefits and blessings of infinite pride and infinite humility simultaneous-

43

ly, infinite solar solipsism and infinite constellation con-
sciousness simultaneously, or whatever else you most desire.
Welcome home, to your perfect paradise on earth!"

Denial, Childishness, and Wavicle Work

Denial, childishness, immaturity, and the "eternal youth" arche-type are the shadow-sides of hopeful innocence and enchant-ment, musical memory, and blissful earthiness and prosperity: all gifts you may be denying yourself if you refuse denial and childishness a legitimate place in your Wholeness.

If you have a wavicle of denial or childishness you may tell it:

"Your denial and childishness are a part of my Wholeness, and I wouldn't be Whole without them. You are my dearly-beloved child, in whom I am well pleased! I love you uncondi-tionally just as you are, and I am here to meet all of your deepest needs, here and now. If you like, you may remain in infinite denial and childishness forever, or if you prefer you may enjoy all the blessings and benefits of infinite denial and infinite acceptance simultaneously, infinite childishness and infinite maturity simultaneously, or whatever else you most desire. Welcome home, to Paradise on Earth!"

Envy, Judgmentalism, and Wavicle Work

Envy, self-righteousness, and cold-hearted judgmentalism are the shadow-sides of compassion, heartfelt care-giving, and lov-ing right-action and justice. If you are denying envy and judg-mentalism as parts of your Wholeness, you may also be denying yourself their gifts.

44

If you encounter a wavicle of envy or self-righteous judgmentalism you may tell it:

"Your envy and judgmentalism are a part of my Wholeness, and I wouldn't be Whole without them. You are my dearly-beloved child, in whom my soul delights! I love you unconditionally and I am here to meet all of your deepest needs, here and now. If you like, you may remain in infinite envy and judgmentalism forever, or if you prefer you may enjoy all the blessings and benefits of infinite envy and infinite care-giving simultaneously, infinite judgmentalism and infinite compassion simultaneously, or whatever else you most desire. Welcome home, to your paradise on earth!"

I once idly wondered what the shadow-side of compassion and care-giving was, and not long afterwards found myself uncharacteristically self-righteous and judgmental of a free-spirited old friend: so intensely judgmental that I had to apologize to him afterwards. I was probably also envious of the very quality I was judging.

I was at a loss to understand where this self-righteous wavicle had come from until I remembered what I had been wondering an hour or two earlier. I learned two lessons that day: what the care-giver's shadow-side was, and that it helps to be consciously aware of what you are asking Creation for, so that when it comes you won't be caught by surprise!

Fear, Flight, and Wavicle Work

Fear, anxiety, and the "bowels turning to water" of terror are the shadow-sides of faithful temperance, liquid belly-laughter, ascension, soaring flight, a quickening of the vibration into the safety of a higher and sacred space, and a radiantly enlightened liberation: all gifts you may be refusing yourself if you refuse to accept fear as an integral part of your Wholeness.

The experience of fear can awaken you from a nightmare into perfect ever-present safety. The same dynamic can apply to actual ascension and dematerialization of your physical body and physical reality in the presence of your luminous Spirit, which like a UFO can induce either terror or ecstasy. Fear is but a form of ecstasy; it can be a quickening which awakens you into safety and freedom.

For a very resistant or fearful wavicle who may appear to be paralyzing us from doing what we must, you may tell it:

"Many thanks for showing me these parts of my Wholeness; I would not be Whole without fear and resistance. I welcome you home unconditionally, just as you are. I love you so much! You are my beloved child in whom I delight! You are free to feel whatever you wish to feel, but I am going to do this thing anyway. If you wish it, I now remind you that you are always unconditionally safe and protected, no matter what it may look like or feel like, for you are eternal, immortal and celestial; you are divine!"

If your wavicle needs safety, you can tell it:

"I give you infinite safety and protection and your own supremely comfortable sacred space; I am here for you, now and always."

If one of your wavicles feels suicidal or wants to die, you can tell it:

"Your desire to die is a part of my Wholeness; I wouldn't be Whole without that flavor, and I thank you for showing it to me so beautifully. I love you unconditionally just as you are. You are free to die into me if you wish. Your desire to die is a divine desire for you to transcend your current limitations and pain. I am so sorry I hurt you for so long. If you wish, with ease, safety, and comfort I release you unconditionally now and forever from all old programs and beliefs of pain, inau-

thenticity, and limitation, and welcome you home into your infinite and eternal freedom. If you wish it, I give you all the divine blessings and benefits of death and all the divine blessings and benefits of eternal life simultaneously, or whatever else you most desire, here in your perfect Heaven on Earth, now and forever."

Please remember that any suicidal thoughts or feelings arising in you always belong to one of your wavicles, not to you as a whole; localize the feeling in your body and do the Wavicle Work on it. If you are feeling gripped by an overwhelming suicidal feeling, please talk to a qualified suicide-prevention counselor immediately. If an *external* wavicle, someone else, expresses suicidal feelings to you, please make sure you put him or her in contact with a qualified suicide-prevention counselor immediately, and then do the Wavicle Work on your internal wavicle represented by that person.

Lust and Wavicle Work

Lust and trespass are the shadow-sides of hopeful generosity, electric sensuality, creative insemination, and blissful passion. If you are rejecting the loving integration of lust and trespass, you may well be denying yourself the gifts of their ripening.

If you are bothered by a lustful wavicle you may tell it:

"Thank you for bringing this to my attention! Your lust and your trespass are part of my Wholeness; I wouldn't be Whole without them! You have done a magnificent job of showing them to me. You may continue in these roles for as long as you like, or if you prefer you may awaken from this wonderful dream of dissatisfaction and come home into your perfect Heaven on Earth, where it is my joy to satisfy all of your deepest desires here and now. If you wish it, I give you all the benefits and blessings of infinite lust and infinite contentment

and fulfillment simultaneously, now and forever. You are my devata, in whom my soul delights! I welcome you home into infinite beauty and love and infinite receptivity for your divinely satisfying blissful passion, now and forever!"

Rebellion and Wavicle Work

Rebellion, cynicism, criticism, and doubt are the shadow-sides of levity, crystal-clarity, bare-bones saturnine simplicity, prudent earthiness, and loving prosperity: all gifts you may be refusing yourself if you refuse to integrate rebellion and criticism into your Wholeness.

If a wavicle is an atheist, or doesn't believe you are really its Creator, or is rebellious, you can tell it:

"Your skepticism, disbelief, rejection, rebellion and doubt are all a part of my Wholeness, and I welcome them and you home, just as you are. You may continue to doubt me forever if you wish, or you may believe in me and rely on me. If you wish I give you all the blessings and benefits of infinite rebellion and doubt and infinitely grounded clarity and simplicity and understanding now and forever. I am sorry I have not consciously been here for you in the past, but I am here for you now and forever; I love you whole-heartedly, and I gladly meet your needs completely and unconditionally; your happiness is my happiness."

If the wavicle still doesn't believe you, you can tell it:

"I give you infinitely satisfying and intelligent proof on the material, sensory level of your justified faith in me and my unconditional support of you forever. I am here to meet your every need; just name it and it is my joy to give it to you, freely and unconditionally, here and now!"

If a wavicle doesn't think having its needs met is realistic, you can tell it:

"All things are possible in me. Just tell me what you need, and I will gladly give it to you. I deal in miracles all the time; I am the creator of your reality."

Humiliation and Wavicle Work

The word *humiliation* comes from the Latin *humilis,* "lowly, humble, on the ground," from *humus,* "earth." Humiliation is feeling like dirt, like a "low-down dirty dog." But dirt and in fact all matter, all of nature, and all creatures are in one sense absolutely and divinely necessary to creation, and on the deepest level, *low-down* and *high-up* are two sides of the same coin; *dirt* is actually *star-stuff*; a *dog* is your best friend and a divine messenger of unconditional love; and Spirit and Matter are One. We would not know Spirit without Matter, and we would not know exaltation without humiliation.

You can tell a humiliated wavicle:

"Thank you so much for showing me this flavor of my Wholeness; I would not be Whole without your humiliation! I love you unconditionally just as you are, and am here to give you whatever you most need. If you like, I give you all the blessings and benefits of infinitely divine humiliation and infinitely divine exaltation simultaneously, now and forever! Welcome home, to your perfect Heaven on Earth."

Guilt and Wavicle Work

Guilt is the shadow-side of responsibility, jovial interdependence, transmutation, radiantly enlightened right-action, and faithful justice, gifts you may be refusing yourself if you refuse to integrate guilt into your Wholeness.

If one of your wavicles feels guilty about wrongdoing, or wants to do the right thing, or doesn't feel it can do the right thing, you can tell it:

"Your guilt is a part of my Wholeness, and I wouldn't be Whole without this guilt. Thank you so much for showing it to me! It is a beautiful dream, and now, if you wish, you may gently awaken to the ever-present truth. You have always been responsible to me; you have always done rightly, and you have always done exactly what I asked you to do. All I have asked of you is that you give me experience, and you have done that perfectly. If you wish it, I give you all the blessings and benefits of guilty wrong-doing and perfect awareness of your infinite right-action and loving justice, simultaneously, now and always."

If a wavicle equates responsibility with heaviness and blame, you can tell it:

"You are responsible only to your highest delight; when you nourish your own light, you nourish the light of all!"

If it doesn't feel deserving, you can tell it:

"Your lack of deservingness is a flavor of my Wholeness and I wouldn't be Whole without it; thank you for showing it to me so perfectly! If you wish it, I now give you all the blessings and benefits of undeservingness together with infinite awareness of your eternal worth and divine deservingness simultaneously; you are my beloved celestial child, in whom my soul delights, now and forever. Welcome home to your perfect Heaven on Earth."

Hurt, Betrayal, and Wavicle Work

Hurt, betrayal, and victimization are the shadow-sides of forgiveness, communion, networking, a "Uranian" or magnetically-flowing liquid sex, and blissful liberation – gifts you may be denying yourself if you refuse to integrate hurt and betrayal as essential parts of your Wholeness. The victim story can be enticing, as it garners sympathy and allows you to feel an interesting drama, but it is ultimately disempowering.

If a wavicle feels hurt and betrayed, you can tell it:

"Thank you for bringing this hurt and betrayal to my attention. Your hurt and betrayal are a part of my Wholeness, and I wouldn't be Whole without these flavors! I love you unconditionally; you are my child in whom my soul delights! I am sorry I hurt you for so long. You may keep all the benefits and blessings of these flavors forever if you like, and if you prefer you may also relax into perfect healing, forgiveness, and divine communion with all of your loved ones, now and forever!"

Confusion and frustration are two more flavors closely related to hurt and betrayal. They tend to arise when a wavicle is entertaining two opposite realities or thoughts simultaneously. You may tell such a wavicle:

"Your confusion and frustration are a part of my Wholeness, and I wouldn't be Whole without them! I love you unconditionally. You are my beloved wavicle-child! Your entertainment of conflicting ideas is part of my Wholeness, for I contain all opposites at once. If you like, I give you all the benefits and blessings of infinite confusion and infinite clarity simultaneously, now and forever, or whatever else you most desire. Welcome home!"

51

Chapter Six

Wavicle Work in Relationships

"Hell is Other People" ... Heaven is Remembering there is only One of Us

Jean-Paul Sartre famously said, "Hell is other people." But as Wavicle Work demonstrates, there really are no other people; there are only wavicles of *you*, expressions of your own infinite consciousness. If you are bothered by someone in your reality, it is often helpful to do the Wavicle Work first on the wavicle closest to you, the one you most identify with, and then work outward from there. Or, simply work on the one that feels the strongest or most intense in this moment.

If you are being bullied by a petty tyrant for example, find the one inside who feels threatened or bullied, and tell that wavicle:

"Your being bullied is a part of my Wholeness; thank you for showing me that flavor! I wouldn't be Whole without it. I love you unconditionally as you are, and am here to give you whatever you most need, now and forever. If you wish it, I freely give you divinely infinite humility and vulnerability and divinely infinite strength and safety and justice, on the tangible level, now and forever. What do you most need?"

When you have given that wavicle everything it needs and it is satisfied, find the bully-wavicle inside of you and tell it:

"Thank you so much for showing me that bullying flavor of my Wholeness! I wouldn't be Whole without it. I love you unconditionally as you are, and I am here to give you whatever you most need, now and forever! What do you most need?"

If it simply needs to feel strong, safe, secure, and happy, just give it that. If it truly needs to dominate, you may wish to give it a whole Universe of its own where it can dominate and rule to its heart's content. You can tell it you will be waiting for it if and when it decides to emerge from that Universe to relate to you as its loving friend and equal.

Soul-Mates

The Soul-Mate is often defined as the one who is God or God-dess incarnate for you, the one who completes you and makes you feel whole. From one point of view, everyone in creation is your Soul-Mate, as they are all incarnations or manifestations of your own Wholeness variously showing you what you most need to see in this moment. And as in your Wholeness you are God or Goddess incarnate for each of your wavicles, you are essentially their perfect Soul-Mate, and hence ultimately your own perfect Soul-Mate, your own divine partner and best friend.

If you find yourself desiring your Soul-Mate, remember this too is the need of a wavicle, and an opportunity to do the seven steps of Wavicle Work for yourself. Once you have localized the wavicle, allowed it to breathe, and welcomed it home as your divine child, you may tell it:

"I give you your perfect soul-mate as your divine lover incar-nate to enjoy heaven on earth with, here, now, and forever!"

This will almost certainly bring up a number of subtle objec-tions from those wavicles who have been following your direc-tives in maintaining your status quo. Integrate them all and your job is done; your divine manifestation is already being drawn to you, from the inside out.

Particle Prayer can also be very useful in attracting your ideal Soul-Mate, here and now. After whole-heartedly imagining and welcoming your supreme God or Goddess, let them approach and embrace you, materializing as your perfect Soul-Mate. Pay close attention to the pleasurable "soul-flavors" or qualities of personality your divine lover shows you; as you appreciate them on the subtle levels, you are "homeopathically" or more accurately "homeo-hedonically" preparing yourself to recognize and accept these gifts in your soul-mate in the physical realm.

The One That Got Away

A sixty-year-old friend once told me he had psychologically been beating himself up for decades for letting the "perfect girl of my dreams" get away when he was a young man. I suggested he find the wavicle who felt that way – he felt it in his heart as an angry, bruised creature – and simply let it breathe and be, and then tell it, *"I give you the perfect girl of your dreams now."*

He felt a little better, but his creature-self then told him it would believe it when it saw the girl physically walk through the door. I suggested he tell the creature, *"I give you the girl of your dreams, physically walking through the door now."*

He felt better still, but then said his creature-self was still feeling bad over having wasted the better part of his life without her. I suggested he tell it, *"you have always made the right choice in any given moment; you are eternally youthful, and I give you an infinite amount of time to satisfy all of your desires."*

As he told his creature-particle this, energy flowed easily throughout his body; his face began to angelically glow, and he looked about forty years younger as he laughed in relief.

It's that simple. The bottom line is, your body believes everything you tell it, both consciously and unconsciously, and will do its best to materialize whatever you are imagining – and its best is very good indeed, for in its own way it is infinitely wiser than you may have been taught to believe. It is actually in simultaneous contact with every other thought-wave and I-particle in creation, and all of these I-particles act in a perfect harmony

54

of divine choreography to play out whatever dramas you require and imagine. In that sense, you could say that every I-particle in creation is a part of your body – your body of awareness, your body of creativity.

If you don't recognize your creation as being the result of your own imagination, you probably have subtler layers of unconscious imaginings operating at cross purposes to your conscious layer of awareness. You can align these layers into coherence by recognizing the perfection of everything. If you are judging anything as not-good, it tends to freeze where it is until you come back and love it unconditionally. By surrendering into Wholeness, you consciously align yourself with your creation. And the more you surrender into Wholeness, the more Wholeness surrenders into you. Like every good marriage, co-creation is a two-way street, with both partners – your imaginative awareness and your body's I-particles – ultimately giving 100%.

Expectation

Notice where you are expecting results from those around you, and remember that everything and everyone is a wavicle of your consciousness. Expectation and its underlying judgment are repulsion-factors. As it says in Al-Anon Family Groups' *Courage to Change*, "An expectation is a premeditated resentment." If you are expecting something from another, you are setting yourself up to feel anger when at some point they inevitably fail to meet your criteria. You are actually disempowering yourself, making your feelings and well-being addictively dependent upon another's actions. The more you judge another, the more you push them away. It's a form of conditional love, not unconditional Love. "I will love you IF…and only IF… you do this for me, or feel this way for me, or act this way for me."

Contrary to what relationship books may teach, successful relationships and genuine intimacy do *not* depend on your communicating every emotion and need to your partner. You may find that the more you attempt to do this, the more your partner runs away, shuts you out, and doesn't return your calls. And sometimes when you play it cool, your partner comes back.

If so, that's not really because you're playing it cool. It's because you have subtly removed your expectations from your partner. That freedom is what brings them back. Intimacy and successful relationships depend on taking up your needs with God, the Wholeness that you are, and getting your wavicle-needs met here and now, and freeing up your partner to enjoy your resulting unconditional Love.

On the other hand, the interior pushing-away or repulsion factor is an integral part of the growth process, as you need to dis-identify with a suffering wavicle, push it out of you, Witness it, and bring it (and you) out of ignorance into "Cosmic Consciousness," before you can communicate with it as its personal Creator, meet its needs, give it the infinitely loving support of "God consciousness," and then bring it into loving alignment and conscious and blissful Unity with you.

100% Responsibility

Please note that this Wavicle Work is to be done internally. The more responsibility you take and unconditional love you give your creation, the more effective Wavicle Work is. You need not get your mate or your parent or your child to learn Wavicle Work in order to make your world better; simply do the Wavicle Work yourself. Your mate, your parent, your child, and everyone in your world, is simply a wavicle of your own infinite consciousness, reflecting some aspect of the One Self. Trying to comb your mirror doesn't work; simply comb your own hair and your reflection automatically improves. Give your inner wavicle what s/he truly needs, and your outer wavicle automatically reflects this change. If they ask, you may share your secret, of course, but it is usually not very efficient or effective to try to get them to do Wavicle Work so that you will feel better.

A friend mentioned she was having trouble with her irresponsible and rebellious son. After learning Wavicle Work and practicing it silently on her "inner son," she returned a few days later and reported that her actual son had immediately become a different person: responsible, well-behaved, loving, and respectful, and that the change appeared to be permanent. This kind of success is delightful to experience, and quite common with Wavicle Work.

Three Stages of Healing

Healing occurs in three stages: First, when you are deeply wounded you naturally suppress; you freeze and stuff the pain down deep, attempting to ignore it. This is traditionally called *tamas* or ignorance (not to be confused with true *Tamas* or dissolution, to be explained later). The suppressed wound is a little like a limb that has fallen asleep. Circulation has effectively bypassed it; the area has gone numb, and you are not consciously aware of it, though the suppressed energies will still "leak" out through unconscious acts and projection.

Second, you act out; you rage or more subtly attempt to give the pain to another in order to get rid of it. This is *rajas* or passion. Acting out is like a sleeping limb that has begun to awaken. As circulation starts to return to it, it prickles like pins and needles. Trying to get the other to change so that you will feel better is akin to this second stage of acting out.

Third, you remain fully aware of the pain, simply letting it *be*, bathing it in unconditional love. This is *sattva* or clarity. Unconditional love is like the full restoration of circulation to the previously-sleeping limb. While all three stages appear to be necessary, Wavicle Work uses this third method; I find it is the only one that really and consistently completes the healing.

Relations with Animals

A friend of mine was plagued by the incessant barking of a neighbor's dog. She decided to try Wavicle Work on it and found the equivalent tension-point in her body, asked it what it needed, and gave it unconditional love, attention, food, and intimacy with its owners on the subtlest finest-feeling level. Almost immediately, the dog stopped barking. Some days later the dog was again barking; she again did the Wavicle Work, this time with a friend, and the dog immediately stopped.

Another friend writes,

"I have two cats, Comedy and Good Buddy. Comedy wouldn't let Good Buddy be friendly. Comedy would hiss at Good Buddy and swat him whenever he came near. It was bothering me. It has been like this since Good Buddy joined the family in September. So I thought, well, if it is all me, then their conflict was mine as well. I did the Wavicle Work of thanking my child for the conflict, finding it in my body, etc. and ended up giving it a friendly relationship where the two cats would play and sleep curled up together and groom each other.

"Two hours later the cats first walked in tandem, then sniffed each other, then licked each other. That night they both slept in the same bed. It has continued [and now] they are good buddies....

"It was so simple!"

Chapter Seven

Wavicle Work in Religion

Reconciliation and Reciprocity

While no religion can be adequately summarized in a few pages, still it appears fair to say that most religions share two fundamental goals: first, to end suffering by *reconciling Spirit (Creator) and Matter (Creation)* through their intermediary, the *conscious Mind or Soul (Creature)*, and second, to spread love and harmony through an *ethic of reciprocity*, known to Christians as the Golden Rule: "Do unto others as you would have them do unto you."

Both reconciliation and reciprocity are easily accomplished with Wavicle Work, which appears to be at the very heart of religion and to be a Mystery immeasurably old, apparently lost and revived many times through the ages. Here are a few traditions in which we can detect the principles of Wavicle Work.

Wavicle Work in the Egyptian Mysteries

In his *Egyptian Light and Hebrew Fire*, Karl W. Luckert emphasizes that Egyptian theology and its offspring Neoplatonism continually highlight the "emanational activity of the godhead as a process of engendering and bringing home." This reconciliation is precisely what you do in Wavicle Work: take responsibility for engendering your wavicles, and bring them home.

Reconciliation of Spirit, Soul, and Matter

Ancient Egyptians in Thebes acknowledged a Holy Family, a Trinity of *Neters* or divine natural principles known as *Amen,*

Mut, and *Khonsu*. *Amen* is the hidden, transcendental, or Heavenly Father, still invoked after prayer. *Mout* or *Mut* is the Earthly Mother; as "Mother Divine" or *Mut Neter* she is remembered as *Mother Nature*. The radiant Child between them is *Khunsu* or *Khonsu*, the divine Son and protector of the king. A younger version of the moon- and magic-god Tahut (Thoth) with whom he was sometimes linked, Khonsu was the lunar "Crosser," the timekeeper, connector, healer, and exorciser of demons. The Theban Trinity beautifully depicts Amen as *Spirit*, Mut as *Matter*, and Khonsu as their intermediary *Soul Consciousness*, their means of reconciliation and healing or making Whole.

Ascending through the Trinity in order of Mother-Son-Father, Mut-Khonsu-Amen, yields the acronym MU-KH-A, meaning "Mouth" or "Face" in Sanskrit. The Egyptian KRST or anointed Christ-body ascended via the ritual of *Opening of the Mouth*, and in Particle Prayer your wavicles ascend through Mother-Matter's Mouth or black hole in love through the singularity of the Son, your radiant Soul-consciousness, and "die" into eternal life by seeing the Face of God the Father, your own blissful white-hole Spirit. A similar term is MOKSHA, "Liberation."

Descending through the Trinity as Father-Son-Mother, Amen-Khonsu-Mut, gives the acronym A-KHO-M, Egyptian for "Hawk" or "Eagle," the sacred birds representing the solar gods Heru or Haru (Horus) and Ra, bringers of life: You descend from Spirit and manifest into Matter in Wavicle Work as *light* and *life*. Akhom, "eagle," is the name of the Coptic letter "A", and so hidden in seed-form in "A" is the entire Trinity, *AKHOM* or *AKHUM*. The Sanskrit Trinity is similarly *AUM*, with "A" for *Brahma(n)* the Creator (cf. *Per-Amen*), "U" for *Vishnu* the Maintainer (cf. *Khunsu*), and "M" for *Shiva* the Destroyer, or more likely his *Shakti* or Goddess-energy, *Mata Devi* (cf. *Mut*): all still present in seed-form in the letter "A", and perhaps all from *AKHUM*. The glottal "A" hieroglyph depicts the Egyptian vulture or Egyptian eagle, symbolizing *Mut*, while the "Akhom" hawk hieroglyph represents a deity or the breast: the "I AM" soul shining in your sacred heart or solar plexus. In Sanskrit, *Aham* is "I". As the "Akhom" hawk represents the solar soul of your solar plexus, and A-KHO-M spans all of creation from

Amen to Mut, your radiantly golden "I AM" consciousness is also the first and the last, or in Greek, the alpha and the omega.

Another form of descent would be Amen-Tahut-Mut, giving the name A-T-M or *Atum*, the Creator-god of Heliopolis, the male-female Wholeness or Father-Mother Cosmic Human (cf. Hebrew *Adam* Kadmon) who begets *Shu* (or *Shwa*) the airy savior-god as the life-bearing phallus-Son (cf. *Yahu-Shwa* and *Shiva*) and *Tefnut* the goddess of order as the moist womb-Daughter (cf. Sanskrit *Devi-nada*, Goddess *Shakti* as divine sound).

The Abydos Trinity was *Ausar* (Osiris) the Father (cf. *Aesir, Asura, Ahura*), *Auset or Eset* (Isis) the Mother, and their child *Ra-Her-Akheti*, the solar Ra-Horus of the Two Horizons as your sacred heart. As the symbol of the solar child is the Eagle or Hawk of Life, *AKHOM*, the Theban Trinity as a whole, so the child, your Consciousness, contains both Father-Spirit and Mother-Matter. Akhenaton identified Ra-Her-Akheti with *Aton* (cf. *Adon, Adonai*), the One male-female God: imageless but symbolized by the sun offering rays with the *Ankh*-cross to your nostrils, showing that the spirit-infused light of your Soul-Consciousness is the one truth, indefinable but uniting all opposites, including "male" Spirit and "female" Matter.

The Memphite Trinity was *P'tah* the Father-Creator (cf. *Pita, Pitar, Pater,* and perhaps *Buddha*), *Sekhmet* the "Powerful Female" Lioness-Mother (cf. *Shekinah, Shakti*, and lion-mounted Durga), and *Nefertem*, the "Lotus of the Sun," the Child. A sculpture of Tut-Ankh-Amen's head emerging from the lotus identifies the young king with Nefertem, the divine Solar Child (Cairo Museum, JE 60723). In earlier versions Nefertem was the son of Nun the god of primeval waters, like Yahushwa, variously translated as Joshua "son of Nun" and Jesus "the Fish."

Egypt also had many other Holy Families of Father, Mother, and Child. All generally represented the trinity of Spirit, Body, and their intermediary offspring Soul, or Consciousness, which emerges from and contains both Spirit-Creator and Matter-Creation as their ultimate reconciliation, as experienced through Wavicle Work.

Pharaoh as Great House and Divine Child

Wavicle Work allows you to easily disidentify with a single soul-wavicle or *Ka* and act as *Pharaoh* – from Ancient Egyptian *Per-aa or Pr-aa*, meaning "Great House" – to your many wavicles, or *Ka*'s. In Egypt, only the pharaoh had a multitude of *Ka*'s, foreshadowing your own mastery as "great house" or container of your creation, where you unite heaven and earth and multiply your single soul-*Ka* into many: like the legendary patriarch Abraham, your wavicle-children as innumerable as the stars in the sky.

Per-aa or *Pr-aa* thus equates to Sanskrit *Brha*, "to grow or multiply:" the root of *Brahm or Brahman*, the emptiful Wholeness, which recalls both *Abraham* of the countless progeny, and the legendary "first pharaoh," *Pr-aa Mn*: Pharaoh *Min* or *Men* ("He who endures"), Greek *Menes*, who united "upper and lower Egypt," heaven's upper chakras with earth's lower chakras. *"Brahman is the eater,"* say the Brahma Sutras; you as primordial pharaoh offer unconditional love to re-member and reintegrate your wavicles, and Khonsu the healer traditionally helps you as pharaoh catch and "eat" or assimilate your wavicles or "other gods," bringing them home into you.

In the Trinity or Holy Family, the Pharaoh often played the part of the Divine Child: whether Nefertem, Ra-Her-akheti, Shu, or Khonsu, always the God the Son mediating between Heavenly Father and Earthly Mother. A lovely limestone sculpture from Karnak shows Tut-Ankh-Amen in Khonsu's place, seated arm-in-arm between Father Amen on his left and Mother Mut on his right, with Amen's right hand on his right shoulder and Mut's left hand on his left shoulder (Cairo Museum CG 4209). As the divine son of the Father and Mother, the god of the Cross reconciling Heaven and Earth, the healer and exorcisor, Khonsu established the god-king Tut-Ankh-Amen as his earthly representative in the Holy Family, seated at the right hand of the Father. Likewise, through Wavicle Work you also mediate between Spirit and Matter to heal and exorcise all your wavicles into harmony and manifest your perfect kingdom of Heaven on Earth.

Identity with the Creator, Creature, or Creation

The Egyptians knew that the Creator-creature kinship is truly one of identity: the Egyptian *Book of Enlightenment* (also known as the *Book of the Coming Forth by Day*, historically the *Book of the Dead*) abounds with statements like "I am Ra" and "I am Ausar (Osiris)" – a wonderful way to align yourself with one or another of your wavicles or devata-names of Wholeness, or God, in order to experience that name's particular divine qualities in the stillness of your own consciousness.

In Wavicle Work, you may play the part of Creator or Father-Spirit to your Mother-Nature or body of creation by attending to your radiant children: your wavicles, creatures, or Souls of Consciousness. In Wavicle Work's other side of Particle Prayer, you play the part of the creature to express the needs of your body of creation or Mother-Nature to your unconditionally loving Father-Spirit. Either way, you are enlivening the same trinity recognized by the Egyptians, reconnecting and reconciling Spirit and Body, or Absolute and Relative, through the wavicles or *Ka*'s of your Soul or Consciousness in order to manifest more and more perfection.

Wavicle Work's "patron saint," Tahut-moses III

The eighteenth dynasty's Pharaoh Thutmose or Tahut-moses III (reigned c. 1490-1436 BCE) was the first person known to claim adoption by a god – *Amen*, the transcendent One, the state God – despite being son of secondary wife Iset (Isis) and not of the Great Queen Hatshetsup, "God's Wife." Upon his adoption by Amen, Tahut-moses III experienced an ascent to Heaven where he was crowned by Ra, the Sun God. As a conscious son of God he became one of history's greatest kings, reigning from Nubia north to the Nile's mouth and across the Near East to the Euphrates River.

Tahut-moses III beautifully exemplifies the Soul's alignment with transcendental Spirit and consequent solar illumination and rulership of Matter: in short, Wavicle Work. Like Tahut-moses III, you too can claim adoption by your Creator, obtain your crown of rulership, and go on to bring all of your countless wavicles into the loving enlightenment of your conscious co-creation.

Pharaoh Tahut-moses III and King David

In his *Christianity: An Ancient Egyptian Religion* (2005), Egyptian scholar Ahmed Osman identifies Pharaoh Tahut-moses III – the Near East's greatest king, ruling from the Nile all the way to the Euphrates – as the legendary King David, said to rule over exactly the same territory. The Egyptian *Tahut* (*TWT*) would in Hebrew be *Da'ud* or *Dawud* (*DWD*), now spelled *David*. Tahut-moses III's divine adoption resonates in King David's Psalm 2:7: *"I will declare the decree: the LORD hath said to me, "You are my son; this day have I begotten you."* What was true for King David is equally true for you and your own wavicles. Whatever your biological ancestry, you can awaken your inner ruler by enlivening your Creator-creature kinship and kingship: the essence of successful Wavicle Work.

David's Hidden Royal Line

Osman believes that Tahut-moses III or King David was the unnamed Biblical pharaoh who met Abraham and his wife Sarai when they came from Ur by way of Canaan to Egypt. When Abraham introduced Sarai to the pharaoh as his sister, Tahut-moses III married and impregnated her, changing her name to Sarah, "Queen." On finding she was Abraham's wife, he returned her to Abraham along with the royal handmaid Hagar to attend to her pregnancy of Isaac.

The story of King David and Uriah's wife Bathsheba is a disguised re-telling of the same drama, as *Uriah* connotes a Yah-worshipper from Ur and *Beth-Sheba* or "daughter of the oath" recalls Abraham's founding of *Beer-Sheba*, the "well of the oath." The Bible repeats the story yet again with Abraham and Abimelech, "Father-King," who took Sarah as Abraham's sister, returned her on finding she was already married, and made a covenant with Abraham at Beersheba: probably agreeing to acknowledge Isaac as his royal progeny. Isaac's grandson Joseph would be prime minister to Pharaoh, and Joseph's grandson would himself be Pharaoh. Likewise your own divinely royal birthright, though perhaps hidden until now, waits for you to claim it and inherit your own kingdom of Heaven on Earth.

Tahut-moses III and Melchizedek

Like every god-king, Pharaoh Tahut-moses III ruled as the upholder of *Ma'at*, variously defined as the *Neter* of cosmic order, divine law, harmony, righteousness, justice, and truth. As *Neb-Ma'at*, the "Lord of Righteousness," his office in Hebrew becomes *Melchizedek*: the "King of Righteousness," the Biblical name of the mysterious *"king of Salem"* and *"priest of the most high God"* who offered bread and wine to Abraham in Genesis 14 and is remembered in Psalm 110, *"The LORD has sworn and will not change his mind: Thou art a priest forever after the order of Melchizedek."*

As a hierophant predating Aaron and offering an archetypal communion to Abraham, the legendary priest-king Melchizedek has inspired countless mystics. Among them was the apostle Paulos or Paul, who described him as, *"Without father, without mother, without descent, having neither beginning of days, nor end of life; but made like unto the Son of God; abideth a priest continually"* (Hebrews 7:3).

According to Osman, Tahut-moses III was Abraham's contemporary and sometime brother-in-law; he would also have been the supreme ruler or king of Salem or Jerusalem, then a territory of Egypt. Before becoming pharaoh he had been trained in the priesthood of Amen, and as the son of Amen and the anointed of Ra, God of the mid-day sun, he was the highest representative on earth of the *"most high God."* Hence he was a divine priest-king and a ruler of righteousness or perfection, a *Neb-Ma'at* or *Melchizedek*, just as you are for your own wavicles.

Tahut-moses III and Hermes Trismegistus

Rosicrucians believe Pharaoh Tahut-moses III founded or restored the Egyptian Mystery School of Tahut or Thoth, Egyptian god of learning and magic. If anything, he probably revived it, as the sphinx, the pyramids, and other highly-advanced artifacts of an antediluvian age suggest that the Egyptian Mysteries of the eighteenth dynasty were remnants of a spiritual science from a sophisticated civilization long predating recorded history. Wavicle Work may actually stem from an ancient Wisdom embracing the sciences of cellular consciousness, electromedicine, fluid vibrations, quantum mechanics, and even the sacred geometry of hyperspace.

Perhaps, then, Tahut-moses III was the (or a) historical figure behind the Greco-Egyptian Hermes Trismegistus: priest, king, and philosopher, and legendary master of the *Hermetic* teachings of *Astrology*, *Alchemy*, and most importantly *Theurgy*, the "divine work" of uniting with God and perfecting one's consciousness: an excellent description of Wavicle Work.

Like Tahut-moses III, Hermes Trismegistus conveyed the Mysteries of Tahut or Thoth, of whom he was said to be an incarnation. Hermes was the Greek form of *Tahut*; *Moses* is Egyptian for "son" or "is born" and Trismegistus means *Thrice-Great*, so that Hermes Trismegistus may well have been Tahut-moses III, "Tahut is born, the *third and greatest.*" Like Tahut-Moses III, Hermes Trismegistus was considered not only a mystery-school founder, but also a contemporary of Abraham.

"Thrice Great" certainly evokes Tahut-moses III's three personas: A *priest* of the spirit like Melchizedek, a *king* of matter like David, and a *philosopher* of the soul like Hermes Trismegistus. And like this thrice-great exemplar, you too can be and eternally are the *priest* or *priestess* of your spiritual Creator, *king or queen* of your material Creation, and *philosopher* for your conscious Creatures, bringing all into harmony with your unconditional love-wisdom in Wavicle Work.

The Emerald Tablet of Hermes Trismegistus

The famed Emerald Tablet of Hermes Trismegistus succinctly summarizes Hermeticism. Molded of green crystal with bas-relief letters in "Syriac" or Phoenician, the original Tablet was reportedly rediscovered in a cavern in the first century CE by the world-teacher Apollonius of Tyana, who then spread its enlightening wisdom everywhere. The Tablet's earliest extant text is a circa-seventh-century Arabic manuscript which was translated into Latin in the twelfth century. It has inspired brilliant minds as diverse as Jabir ibn Hayyan ("Geber"), Albertus Magnus, Roger Bacon, Johannes Trithemius, Michael Maier, John Dee, Isaac Newton, Aleister Crowley, and C. G. Jung.

Isaac Newton translates it thus: *"1. 'Tis true without lying, certain & most true. 2. That which is below is like that which is above & that which is above is like that which is below to do the miracles of one only thing. 3. And as all things have been & arose from one by the mediation of one: so all things have their birth from this one thing by adaptation. 4. The Sun is its father, the moon its mother, the wind hath carried it in its belly, the earth is its nurse. 5. The father of all perfection in the whole world is here. 6. Its force or power is entire if it be converted into earth. 7. Separate thou the earth from the fire, the subtle from the gross sweetly with great industry. 8. It ascends from the earth to the heaven & again it descends to the earth & receives the force of things superior & inferior. 9. By this means you shall have the glory of the whole world 10. & thereby all obscurity shall fly from you. 11. Its force is above all force. For it vanquishes every subtle thing & penetrates every solid thing. 12. So was the world created. 13. From this are & do come admirable adaptations whereof the means (or process) is here in this. Hence I am called Hermes Trismegist, having the three parts of the philosophy of the whole world. 14. That which I have said of the operation of the Sun is accomplished & ended."*

The Emerald Tablet is a wonderful exposition of Wavicle Work. It describes the quantum, holo-fractal nature of Wholeness (lines 1-3); it shows how unifying your fiery solar spirit and watery lunar body with your airy breath (wind) will manifest your quintessential soul-consciousness of earthly perfection (lines 4-6), via the subtlest-feeling-level technique of withdrawing your senses and engaging in Creator-creature dialogue (lines 7-8); it gives the enlightening results (lines 9-10), and it summarizes Wavicle Work's ultimate spirit-soul-body creativity (lines 11-13) and achievement of the Great Work (line 14).

The Egyptian Arts of Astrology and Alchemy

Of the three Hermetic sciences, Wavicle Work begins with the divine work of Theurgy, of uniting with God, but also embraces the heights of Astrology and depths of Alchemy. That the Ancient Egyptians were expert at astrology from ages past is manifest in their sacred texts and the stellar alignments of the sphinx and of the Giza pyramids, which appear to reflect the three stars of the Belt of Orion, who assisted the Pharaoh to ascend to the stars, and which may be linked to both Sirius and the Draco constellation as well. All of these stars are also wavicles in your Wholeness, children of your own consciousness. If misused, astrology can promote fatalistic defeatism, but used properly it can serve as a beautiful form of Wavicle Work. By acknowledging inchoate feelings and then localizing them into specific planetary aspects or wavicles within your zodiacal chart or your "body of awareness," you can lovingly integrate them into harmony with you.

Alchemy also apparently originated in Ancient Egypt; its very name stems from the Arabic *Al-khem*, "the Egyptian" art. *Khem* means not only "Egyptian" but also "black," for Egypt's dark, fertile earth; black also symbolized rebirth. Properly applied, internal alchemy transmutes your body of awareness through the Dark Night of the Soul into crystalline or golden perfection, and thereby uncovers the immortality of the eternal present within the mercurial nature of your own primordial bliss-consciousness. With Wavicle Work you easily accomplish this by transmuting the darkest lead of your "demonic" suffering into the brightest gold of your divine love.

The Egyptian Golden Rule

Wavicle Work's golden love is both practiced inwardly and manifested outwardly through the Golden Rule: do unto others (your wavicles, both inner and outer) what you would have done to you. The Golden Rule in Egypt dates back at least 650 years before Tahut-moses III to the Middle Kingdom, c. 2100 B.C., as evinced in the tale of *The Eloquent Peasant*: "Now this is the command: Do to the doer to cause that he do thus to you." This is a perfect description of the "instant-feedback" principle of Wavicle Work: whatever you do to "others" or to your devatas, causes them to do the same to you, for you are actually doing it to wavicles of yourself. This instant feedback is the Grace of Wholeness nudging you to take full responsibility for your creation.

Other Egyptian Exemplars of Wavicle Work

Some other inspiring Egyptian exemplars of Wavicle Work include many of the "Golden Age" eighteenth-dynasty god-kings and queens descending from the proposed historical model for King David, Melchizedek, and Hermes Trismegistus: Tahut-moses III, both through his grandson and namesake, Tahut-moses IV of the famous Dream Stele, and eventually through Isaac, his son by Sarah and the stepson of Abraham.

Amenhotep III

Tahut-moses IV and his wife Mut-em-wiya had Amen-hotep III, "the Magnificent" (ruled c. 1405-1367 BCE), a supremely wealthy, wise, and powerful king whom Osman identifies as the original, historical King Solomon. His name means "Amen is at peace," which in Hebrew would be Salom-amen, written SLMMN, and his (Amen-em-opet's) *Book of Wisdom* is often compared to Solomon's *Proverbs*. Like Solomon, he inherited an enormous empire reaching from the Nile to the Euphrates and ruled it peacefully by organizing it into 12 zodiacal administrative districts, each supplying taxes to support the kingdom for one month of the year; he built the walls and earthwork of Jerusalem along with the royal cities of Megiddo, Hazor, Gezer, and a network of far-flung military outposts; he developed chariots as a separate wing of the army; he enjoyed a large harem including numerous foreign princesses and the "Pharaoh's daughter" (a privilege actually reserved only for Egyptians), and he erected enormous temples and a royal palace complex as described in the Bible. Egyptian culture and commerce flourished in an unprecedented Golden Age under this master of Wavicle Work and cosmic administration.

Tiye

Amenhotep III's favorite wife Tiye was daughter of his prime minister, Yuya, the immensely influential and wealthy foreign "father to Pharaoh" who Osman affirms was the historical Joseph the Patriarch, grandson of Isaac and great-grandson of Tahut-moses III and Sarah. By marrying Amenhotep III and birthing Akhenaton, identified by Osman as the historical Moses, the powerful Tiye would reunite the two lines of Tahut-moses III or King David. Perhaps influenced by Tiye, Amenhotep III promoted the worship of the imageless Aton, even calling himself *Aton tjehen*, "the dazzling sun-disk," while acknowledging Amen and all other gods in peaceful tolerance. As Solomon he is also credited with a great Mystery School, perhaps perpetuating the Wavicle Work insights of his ancestor, Tahut-moses III or David, supplemented by Tiye's Atonist wisdom.

Tiye's exquisite Nubian features recall the bride in the Song of Solomon, who is *"black, but comely"* and compared to *"a company of horses* [or *"my mare"*] *in Pharaoh's chariots,"* hinting at her father Yuya's position as commander of Amenhotep's chariots. Amenhotep III was crowned upon marrying Tiye, and the Song of Solomon reads, *"... behold king Solomon with the crown wherewith his mother crowned him the day of his espousals, and in the day of the gladness of his heart."* (Song of Solomon, 1:5-9; 3:11.) Their royal wedding and his coronation would reenact the divine marriage of heavenly Amen and earthly Mut and the rebirth of Khonsu, celebrated at the Opet Festival near the fall equinox.

Ram and Sita?

Amen-hotep III's throne name was Neb-Maat-*Ra* or "Righteous King Ra;" if he was indeed Moses' father, he was also the Biblical Am*ram* (Amen-Ra?). As his Great Royal Wife was "the pharaoh's daughter" *Sita*men, it is tempting also to see the Vedic righteous Solar King *Ram* and his beloved *Sita* in this couple: Though their stories now differ in many details, both kings were renowned for their solar wisdom and presided over a golden age; both were involved in exile (Amenhotep III's was really his son's, but King Solomon also reportedly spent time in exile), and both Solomon and Ram were legendary masters of demons: again, exemplars of Wavicle Work, which turns your suffering demons into your blissful devotees.

Akhenaton

Amen-hotep III and Tiye had Amen-hotep IV (co-regent c. 1378 BCE; ruled alone c. 1367-1361 BCE), who married Kiya and the famous Nefertiti. On obtaining the throne he changed his name to Iakh-en-Aton or Akhenaton ("Shining Spirit of Aton"), which appears in the Bible with the key elements transposed as *Adoniyah* or *Adonijah*. He established a new holy capital as his "Eden" at Akhet-Aton ("Horizon of Aton," modern Amarna; cf. *Echad Adon*, "One God"), where he and Nefertiti would offer flowers, unguents, incense, and 12 loaves of showbread to the imageless Aton. Their One God was shown as a sun-disk with rays offering ankh-crosses of divine life-breath to the nostrils of the pharaoh's family: a perfect illustration of the use of breath in Wavicle Work to unite Spirit and Body.

Reacting against their powerful priesthoods, Akhenaton then rejected Amen and all the other gods, destroyed their images, closed their temples, and dispossessed their priests: eventually sparking a counter-revolution banishing him and his court. Ahmed Osman believes that as the first iconoclastic monotheist who led his followers on an Exodus out of Egypt, Akhenaton was the historical Moses. Ralph Ellis (*Eden in Egypt*) feels that Akhenaton was both Adam and Aaron, while his brother Tahutmoses, about whom very little is known, was actually Moses. But Akhenaton did claim to be the only son (or "Moses") of God, while also depicting himself as a nude hermaphrodite, like the male-female Atum or Adam Kadmon, the cosmic Man. He and his family often appeared nude or nearly nude in his garden paradise. He was expelled from "Eden" because he partook of the "Tree of Knowledge of Good and Evil" by rejecting Amen

71

and the other gods of his ancestors, and he plucked their divine names from the "Tree of Life" where Tahut traditionally inscribed them, depriving them of eternal life by erasing all of their sacred inscriptions. If Akhenaton was "Adam," his original sin was not carnal knowledge but dualistic intolerance.

Scholars Messod and Roger Sabbah (*Secrets of the Exodus: Egyptian Origins of the Hebrew People*) place the Exodus a generation later, believing that Moses was pharaoh Ra-Moses I (ruled c. 1335-1333 BCE) and Joshua was Seti I (Hebrew Shadai; ruled c. 1333-1304 BCE), who reconquered Palestine for Egypt and planted the monotheistic followers of Akhenaton there as a buffer colony. Osman's model rings true spiritually while the Sabbahs' model makes sense politically; perhaps both are true, and several generations were later conflated into one.

Whether or not he was the historical Moses, Akhenaton directly impacted Judaeo-Christianity. He was the first exclusive monotheist; his beloved god Aton remains as Adon and Adonai; his Great Hymn resonates in Psalm 104, and metallurgist Robert Feather (*The Mystery of the Copper Scroll at Qumran: The Essene Record of the Treasure of Akhenaten*) proves Akhenaton was the root-progenitor of the Essenes, as evidenced by their Egyptian-copper scroll listing his treasures and their reverent memory of Akhenaton's Temple at Akhet-Aton. His imageless One God, Aton, beautifully expresses Wholeness uncolored by any specific wavicle.

Tut-Ankh-Amen

Ahmed Osman believes Akhenaton's successor Tut-Ankh-Aton ("Living Image of Aton," ruled c. 1361-1352 BCE) appears in the Bible as Moses' successor Yahushwa, variously translated as Joshua, Iesous, or Jesus: *Joshua* (from the Hebrew) and *Jesus* (from the Greek) were originally used interchangeably in the Bible for the same person, appearing *physically* with Moses on the mount (described in Exodus 24 and implied in Matthew 17), and *spiritually* to the Apostle "Paulos" or Paul some 1400 years later.

Called the living image of God from birth, when he was crowned at age nine he became the divine king through anointing by fat of the "dragon" or crocodile: *Meseh* in Egyptian, the root of the word *Messiah*, the anointed one, in Greek the *Christos*. As god-king in the flesh he assumed the role of Khonsu-Tahut, Shu, and Nefertem: divine child and intermediary between Heaven and Earth, healer, exorcisor of demons, savior, and the Solar Son of Nun (god of primeval waters); and in the spirit he is also the Fish, Lord of the Piscean Age.

From childhood Tut-Ankh-Aton and his wife Ankh-es-en-pa-Aton worshipped the One Aton, but after gaining the throne he revived the traditional Egyptian Mysteries. He changed his name to Tut-Ankh-*Amen* ("Living Image of Amen"), resanctified and restored the desecrated temples of Amen-Ra – thus "ejecting the moneychangers" from them – and reinstated all of the other gods and their priests. Osman interprets Yeshaiyahu or Isaiah 7:14, written about the Messiah in the 8th century BCE, as history rather than prophecy: *"Therefore, the Lord himself gives you a sign: Behold, a virgin* [or *"young woman"*] *conceives, and calls his name Immanuel,"* i.e., *Amen-u-El:* "Amen is his God."

Tut-Ankh-Amen died at about nineteen. Following Jewish texts, Osman suggests he was slain for his spiritual "idolatry" or "adultery" and hanged on a tree by Akhenaton's "wicked priest" Panehesy or Phinehas, while on an ecumenical mission to reunify the Amenists and Atonists with Aton as the Supreme God and the other gods as Aton's "angels" or "saints" or wavicles: an approach that early Christianity took with much success.

Robert Feather (*Secret Initiation of Jesus at Qumran*) shows that Christian Copts later re-used Panehesy's empty tomb as a chapel, actually painting a haloed baby Jesus into the arms of the original mural's Nefertiti, who was Tut-Ankh-Amen's mother or stepmother. The cross of the crucifixion was unknown in early Christian art; the earliest form of cross depicted was the Copts' Egyptian Ankh, the cross of eternal life central to the name of Tut-*Ankh*-Amen.

After his violent death, Tut-Ankh-Amen was buried in another's rock-cut tomb, anointed and in raiment nearly identical to that of a Jewish high priest, with funeral furniture resembling the Tabernacle and the Ark of the Covenant, along with a beautiful alabaster jar of perfume and a gilded throne showing his wife lovingly anointing him under the 12 rays of Aton. (She too had changed her name, from Ankh-es-en-pa-*Aton* to Ankh-es-en-*Amen*, but she was certainly his *Mery*, his "beloved.") Some of his burial statues wore vestments like Christian dalmatics and miters; one had a crozier like a bishop's, and a painting on his tomb-wall depicted Tut-Ankh-Amen in triune form as divine Father (Osiris), Son (Horus), and "Holy Ghost" (Ka).

In *Tutankhamun: The Exodus Conspiracy* (2010), Andrew Collins and Chris Ogilvie-Herald relate that upon discovering Tut-Ankh-Amen's tomb in 1922, Howard Carter and his patron Lord Carnarvon found papyri which Carter asked philologist Sir Alan Gardiner to help translate. Carter later threatened to publish their contents as the true history of the Exodus: a potential bombshell, as delicate negotiations were then underway to restore Palestine to the Jews. The papyri, if any, remain hidden to this day.

Why the name *Yahushwa*? The Sabbahs (*Secrets of the Exodus*) suggest that the Midianites' *Yahu* was a title of their god-king: Tut-Ankh-Amen's grandfather, Amen-hotep III, and passed down through his heirs. *Yah* was also a name for the Moon-God Khonsu-Tahut, who was often identified with both Amenhotep III and Tut-Ankh-Amen. And Khonsu-Tahut was sometimes linked with *Shu* (or perhaps *Shwa*), who lifts up the deceased to heaven and offers the life-breath as the savior-god. It is this life-breath that you use in Wavicle Work to localize, witness, and heal your suffering wavicles.

Shu is the divine Son of *Atum* the male-female Creator and cosmic Man (as in *Adam* Kadmon); in Hebrew, the Son of *Adam* is literally the Son of *Man*. And Khonsu is also the great serpent who fertilizes the cosmic egg. As John 3:14 says, *"And as Moses lifted up the serpent in the wilderness,"* the serpent being the Pharaoh's staff, one's inner *kundalini*, and Khonsu, *"even so must the Son of Man* [literally, *"Son of Adam"*] *be lifted up."* This verse hints at Moses as Atum/Adam the creator, lifting up the cosmic serpent as his divine son Khonsu/Yah-Shu.

Perhaps *Yahu* comes ultimately from the Egyptian *Iakhu*, meaning "Shining," "Spirit," or "Manifesting." Yahushwa might then derive from an Egyptian *Iakhu-Shu* (or *Iakhu-Shwa*), a radiant Sun God who descends, incarnates, and manifests, and then ascends as Son and savior; both names appear together on an ancient Egyptian Coffin text (VI,89e, f): *"It is on Shu that I have gone up; it is on Iakhu that I have gone down."* Jewish texts also refer to an earlier messiah named Yeshua ben *Pandera*, the Hebrew rendition of the Egyptian *Pa-neter-Ra*, the Sun God. If *Iakhu* appears in *Iakh*-en-Aton, *Iakhu-Shwa* could perhaps be the *Shu* or son of Akhenaton/Moses, who by also depicting himself as Atum/Adam the First Man, the Cosmic Human, would fall or descend in order to rise again as the Son of Man.

By any name, the young god-king was the last branch *("Netzer,"* hence *"Nazarene")* of the great royal tree of Tahut-moses III or King David, but the beautiful vision of tolerance which Osman ascribes to him lives forever and is the essence of Wavicle Work, which sees every being as a divine wavicle of your Wholeness or Aton. His ancestral Mystery School's healing principles of Wavicle Work may have survived through the Alexandrian Therapeuts and the Essenes of Qumran and Mt. Carmel, and into the present Age via the Gnostics' Apostle "Paulos" or Paul of Tarsus. "Paulos" may actually have been "Apollos" or Apollonius of Tyana, the first-century Neo-Pythagorean master who reportedly rediscovered the Emerald Tablet of Hermes Trismegistus, comprehended it fully, and traveled throughout the known world, including Tarsus, Antioch, Corinth, and Rome, reviving the various Mysteries and restoring forgotten sacred rites in the loving spirit of Tut-Ankh-Amen.

Wavicle Work in Wicca

Founders of Wicca

Wicca as a formal religion is relatively new, but its inspiration is age-old. The "Grandmother of Wicca" would be the famed English Egyptologist and archeologist Margaret Murray (1863-1963), who studied and taught with Sir Flinders Petrie from 1894 and excavated with him in Egypt from 1902 until its Ottoman rulers allied with the Germans in World War I. By then she had written numerous works including grammars on Ancient Egyptian (1905) and Coptic (1911), and most recently an article on "Evidence for the Custom of Killing the King in Ancient Egypt" for *Man* in 1914.

Murray then turned to local folklore, writing two pieces on "The Egyptian Elements in the Grail Romance" for *Ancient Egypt* in 1916. Upon researching the European witch trials, Murray wrote several articles suggesting that witches represented the remnants of an ancient Pre-Christian fertility religion. While maintaining her life-long study of Egypt – she was Assistant Professor of Egyptology at the University College of London from 1924 to 1935 – she wrote her seminal *The Witch-Cult in Western Europe* in 1921, followed by the article on "Witchcraft" for the *Encyclopedia Britannica* (1929), which remained in print for 40 years, and *The God of the Witches* in 1931 (reissued 1952). In 1954 she wrote *The Divine King in England,* asserting that ritual king-killing had survived into early modern times. That year she also wrote the introduction to *Witchcraft Today* by Gerald Gardner (1884-1964), the acknowledged "Father of Wicca."

Though Margaret Murray's witchcraft studies were widely criticized as biased and flawed by scholars, they nevertheless ignited the imaginations of many, including Gerald Gardner, who had joined the Rosicrucian Order Crotona Fellowship and the New Forest Coven in the 1930s, and founded his own Bricket Wood Coven in the 1940s. When England repealed its Witchcraft Laws in 1951, Gardner went public, promoting a new, nonviolent form of the "oldest religion" worldwide. Gardnerian Wicca attempted to revive the Mysteries by combining traditional coven rituals with Freemasonry and ceremonial magic, which in turn derive in part from Hermetic and Ancient Egyptian sources. From the original Gardnerian, Wicca has since developed many other traditions, including Alexandrian, Algard, Dianic, Seax, Celtic, Egyptian, Faery, Norse, and Solitary.

Reconciliation in Wicca

Wicca is a neo-Pagan, earth-centered religion, acknowledging the essential unity of spirit and matter. Wiccans generally gather in covens no larger than thirteen to celebrate the seasons with solar *Sabbat* rites at the solstices, equinoxes, and cross-quarters, and lunar *Esbat* rites at the full moons. Some branches of Wicca celebrate "sky-clad" or nude, while others wear ceremonial robes. Wiccans today are highly individualistic and acknowledge no central authority or dogma, but many affirm an indescribable One-ness or Wholeness which manifests into duality as a God and Goddess like Osiris (or Serapis) and Isis: sometimes envisioned as the male Horned God of the hunt or Sacrificial God of vegetation, the Lord of the life force, or the Sun; and the female Great Mother or Triple Goddess of Maiden, Mother, and Crone, the Lady of material creation, or the Moon.

Wiccan ritual aligns the practitioners through the High Priestess and High Priest with the Goddess and God, and as such is essentially Theurgy, what we would call a form of the Particle Prayer of Wavicle Work. Many Wiccans celebrate God's marriage to Goddess symbolically with the "Grail Hallows" of blade and chalice; a couple may also celebrate the Great Rite physically with sexual intercourse. Whether symbolically or physically, uniting the solar male and lunar female is a form of reconciliation of spirit and matter. In addition, most Wiccans practice Magic to align with their divine Creator and then to manifest their deepest, truest, most divine purpose through co-creation: in essence, the art of Wavicle Work.

Some Wiccans also practice the Hermetic Arts of astrology and alchemy (particularly plant alchemy), and Wicca itself has adopted the Hermetic and Pythagorean pentagram or pentalpha as its symbol, taking its five points to symbolize the four elements of matter (earth, air, water, and fire) with the fifth or quintessence being spirit, thus another expression of the reconciliation and essential unity of matter and spirit. The pentagram contains three different examples of *phi* or the golden ratio, present everywhere in nature and held sacred by the Ancient Egyptians who incorporated it into the pyramids.

Wiccan practitioners of Magic often open and close a ritual by making the sign of the pentagram at each of the four quarters. Advanced Wavicle Work archetypal studies reveal a curious pattern of four interlocking pentacles marking 24 specific High Feasts throughout the Solar Calendar year, with one point of each pentagram opening to an equinox or solstice and the other four points in signs of each of the four elements.

Reciprocity in Wicca

Modern Wiccans unanimously adhere to the Wiccan Rede: *"An* [meaning *"if"*] *it harm none, do as ye will."* The unwillingness to harm anything is the ultimate expression of the negative form of the Golden Rule, or what is known as the Silver Rule: "Do not do unto others what you would not wish done to yourself."

Most Wiccans also believe in the Rule of Three, which states that whatever energy you put out into the world is returned to you three-fold, so they are careful to do only good: yet another expression of the Golden Rule and the "instant-feedback" of Wavicle Work: what you do to "others," you actually do to yourself, as all "others" are actually wavicles of your own consciousness, through whom you "magically" experience the effects of your own creation.

Other Wiccan Exemplars of Wavicle Work

In addition to Margaret Murray and Gerald Gardner, some of the many other inspiring exemplars of Wicca and the magic of Wavicle Work (with some of their books) are Doreen Valiente (*The Charge of the Goddess, The Rebirth of Witchcraft, Natural*

Magic, An ABC of Witchcraft Past and Present, Witchcraft for Tomorrow), Alex Sanders (*Lectures, Book of Law*), Janet and Stewart Farrar (*The Witches' Goddess, The Witches' God, A Witches' Bible*), Raymond Buckland (*The Tree: Complete Book of Saxon Witchcraft, Buckland's Complete Book of Witchcraft*), Scott Cunningham (*Wicca: A Guide for the Solitary Practitioner*); Starhawk (*The Spiral Dance*), Shadwynn (*The Crafted Cup*), and Ellen Cannon Reed (*The Witches' Qabalah, Circle of Isis: Ancient Egyptian Magic for Modern Witches*).

Wavicle Work in Judaism

King David and Wavicle Work

One of the greatest exponents of Wavicle Work was the legendary King David, a brilliant warrior who ruled "from the River of Egypt to the great river, the river Euphrates" (Genesis 15:18). Had he only conquered the known world, King David would not really merit notice here, but he is also credited with authoring the Psalms, among which is the crown-jewel of divine adoption found in Psalm 2:7-8: *"I will declare the decree: the LORD hath said to me, "You are my son; this day have I begotten you. Ask of me, and I shall give you the heathen for your inheritance, and the uttermost parts of the earth for your possession."* David awakens your inner ruler by enlivening your creature-Creator kinship and Creator-creation kingship: the essence of successful Wavicle Work. You can say something like this to your own wavicles, telling them that they are your children, and if they ask it, you will give them an entire world.

The Creator communicates powerfully to the creature in King David's Psalm 46:10, *"Be still (or "Let go," "Let be," "Surrender"), and know that I am God. I will be exalted among the nations; I will be exalted in the earth."* It is by being still and letting go that your internal "wars cease to the ends of the earth." When you as creature surrender into the unconditional love of the Creator, your Creator-Self blesses your creature-self with unconditional love to peacefully rule your creation. You may not experience yourself to be the Creator of everything, but you are made in the Creator's image and likeness (Genesis 1:26), and you are certainly the Creator of your inner thought-wavicles. And you can say something like this to your own wavicles, *"Relax, and know that I am your Creator; I am taking care of you, and of everyone!"*

David says in Psalm 82:6-8, *"I have said, You are gods, and all of you are children of the most high. But you shall die like men (or "like Adam"), and fall as one of the princes. Arise, O God; judge the earth, for you shall inherit all nations."* When your princely intellect, a divine wavicle-child of your Wholeness, perceives it has been seeking the eternal in the ephemeral, it surrenders its strife and falls or "dies" into its divine inheritance, your own Wholeness; and as Wholeness you then arise, judge the earth, and everywhere find only your own Wholeness therein. Whatever you give your wavicles, you experience for yourself; why not give them perfection?

King Solomon and Wavicle Work

Inheriting King David's enormous empire from the Nile to the Euphrates was King Solomon, another exemplar of Wavicle Work. A legendary king of enormous wisdom, wealth, and power, as well as a great lover of pleasure, Solomon ruled peacefully through skillful diplomacy and judicious marriage to the beautiful royal daughters of many of his neighboring rulers. Perhaps influenced by a favorite wife, he promoted the worship of the imageless *Adon* or *Adonai*, while also honoring the other gods in what we now see as a beautiful understanding of Wavicle Work, wherein the indefinable Wholeness has many divine wavicles, and in fact every being is a divine expression of the One Wholeness.

Psalm 72:1 reads, *"A Psalm for Solomon: Give the King your judgments, O God, and your righteousness unto the King's son."* This psalm recalls the mysterious *Melchizedek*, Hebrew for the "King of Righteousness," the Biblical name of the mysterious "King of Salem," literally, the King of Peace, the unifier of Heaven and Earth and enjoyer of that unified perfection. You are the Melchizedek for your wavicles, unifying Spirit and Matter in unconditional love, peace, and perfection.

Midrash Ecclesiastes Rabbah (7:23 No. 1) states also that King Solomon was an expert in astrology. As we have seen, astrology is one of the three Hermetic sciences, and is an opportunity to practice wavicle work by localizing abstract issues into specific planetary or stellar wavicles which we can then integrate in unconditional love.

The Song of Solomon is a beautiful paean to the sacred marriage of Heaven and Earth, or Spirit and Matter: he, whose skin is as gold, ivory, and marble (5:14-15), and she, who is "black, but comely" (1:5). When you unify Spirit and Matter by blessing your wavicles or subtle senses, the natural result is exquisite celestial pleasure.

Moses and Wavicle Work

A prince of Ancient Egypt, *Moses* (Egyptian for "son" or "born," or Hebrew for "drawn out") was Judaism's most important prophet and teacher, credited for leading the Israelites on their Exodus out of Egypt, communing with YHWH, bringing the Ten Commandments to his people, and writing the Torah or Pentateuch.

Just as Moses drew the Israelites out of bondage to the promised land of milk and honey, so you too can free your unhappy wavicles, who have been bound in servitude to beliefs of lack and limitation, into a world of infinite abundance and perfection.

Moses' iconoclastic and monotheistic insistence on the One God, *Adon* or *Adonai*, who is beyond all images and forms, is a beautiful honoring of your own Wholeness, uncolored by any wavicle, and a reminder to use Wavicle Work to disidentify yourself from any wavicle or "idol" that is causing you suffering. At the same time, his conception of God as a supreme being who cares about you is an inspiring call both to play the part of the creature to your Creator through Particle Prayer, and to transmit that same caring to your own wavicles or creatures as their loving Creator, as you are made in the Creator's image and likeness.

Yahushwa and Wavicle Work

Yahushwa, meaning *"Yahu is salvation,"* is translated variously from the Hebrew as Yeshua or Joshua and from the Greek as Iesous or Jesus, and appears first in the Torah as the son of Nun and successor of Moses, and second in Zechariah 6:11 as the son of Yahuzedek ("Yahu is righteousness"), and as the priest-king who is crowned as the Branch and builder of the Temple. The *Branch* recalls Yeshaiyahu or Isaiah 4:2, *"In that day shall the branch of the Lord be beautiful and glorious, and the fruit of the earth shall be excellent and comely for them that are escaped of Israel."* Isaiah also says that *"out of the stem of Jesse* [David's father] ... *a Branch* [Hebrew *"Netzer"*] *shall grow out of his roots"* (Isaiah 11:1). Jeremiah, too, speaks of the *"righteous Branch"* growing from David's line to *"execute judgment and righteousness in the land"* (Jeremiah 23:5, 33:15).

Like Yahushwa, you too are in essence a *Netzer* or Branch of the Creator's adoption, extending the blessings of unconditional love and "righteousness" or perfection to those wavicles which you (like Moses) have delivered from bondage, and offering them all the excellent and comely fruits of the earth. Your body of creation is the gloriously holy Temple you are building in which all of your wavicles may enjoy the harmony of love and devotion in the One Wholeness in Heaven on Earth.

Judaism and Theurgy

Judaism expresses the mysteries of reconciliation of Spirit and Matter in the *Merkabah* and the *Kabalah*, two forms of Theurgy. The Merkabah (or Vector Equilibrium Matrix) is Ezekiel's "chariot of ascension" and "throne of God," which is thought to be an Egyptian term invoking the subtle-body's pyramid of light or *Mer* to raise the soul or *Ka* to the spirit or *Ba*. The related mysteries of the *Kabalah* use the "Tree of Life" of ten planetary Sephiroth or Archetypes linked by 22 paths to depict the sequential stages of emanation from the Godhead to Earth, and to provide a specific path of ascension back to the source.

The Kabalistic Jewish teaching of *Tikkun 'Olam* or "healing the world" states that the perfection of the world is in your hands; there is no one else to do it but you: a call to take 100% responsibility for your world as in Wavicle Work, where you heal your entire world and everyone in it into the perfection of unconditional love.

Judaism, Astrology and Alchemy

While Judaism has long been ambivalent about astrology, the Tosefta (Kiddushin 5:17) affirms that the Lord's blessing on Abraham, making his descendants as numberless as the stars in the sky (Genesis 22:17), was the gift of astrology. It is also a beautiful description of your own wavicles. Scholars have seen astrological references in the 12 sons of Jacob, the 12 tribes of Israel, the 12 loaves of show-bread and the 12 stones of the High Priest's breastplate as representing the 12 signs of the zodiac; the seven branches or "lights" of the Menorah as representing the seven classical "planets," Sun, Moon, Mercury, Venus, Mars, Jupiter, and Saturn, each of which still rules a day of the week; and Ezekiel's four "living creatures" of the Merkabah or chariot-throne of God as the fixed signs of the zodiac: human for Aquarius, ox for Taurus, lion for Leo, and eagle for Scorpio (Ezekiel 1:10). All of these astrological elements represent healing tools and techniques used in the sacred geometry of advanced Wavicle Work.

The fourth-century Egyptian alchemist Zosimos credited his learning to Mary the Jewess, and said the Jews had gained the secrets of the "sacred craft" of Alchemy from the Egyptians and then transmitted the knowledge of the "power of gold" to the rest of the world. Wavicle Work employs internal Alchemy to establish mastery of this "power of gold," both as the golden light of loving reconciliation, and the Golden Rule of loving reciprocity with your wavicles or "children."

Judaism gives the Golden Rule in Leviticus 19:18: *"You shall not avenge, nor bear any grudge against the children of your people, but you shall love your neighbor as you love yourself. I am the Lord."* And not just your own people: *"But the stranger who dwells with you shall be as one born among you, and you shall love him as yourself, for you were strangers in the land of Egypt. I am the Lord your God."* (Leviticus 19:34). The great Rabbi Hillel the Elder (c. 110 BCE – 10 CE) beautifully expresses the negative version of the Golden Rule, commonly known as the Silver Rule, as follows: "That which is hateful to you, do not do to your fellow. That is the whole Torah; the rest is the explanation; go and learn."

Other Jewish Exemplars of Wavicle Work

In addition to King David, King Solomon, Moses, and Yahushwa, some of the most inspiring Jewish exemplars of Wavicle Work include the Therapeuts of Alexandria, the Essenes of Qumran and Mt. Carmel, Hillel the Elder, Philo of Alexandria, Akiva ben Joseph, Simeon bar Yochai, Moses de Leon, and Baruch Spinoza, who understood the unity of spirit and matter as a single "substance" (or Wholeness), of which every lesser entity is a modification (or wavicle), along with the inherent perfection of reality.

Wavicle Work in Christianity

Spiritual Reconciliation

The spiritual reality of Jesus or Yahushwa the Nazarene, the *Netzer* or "Branch" of King David, and the *Meshiah* or *Christos*, the anointed Messiah, has been felt by countless millions for millennia and serves as a profound line of Spirit-Matter reconciliation, or Initiation into Wholeness. Christians have always connected Yahushwa not only to the line of King David, who claimed sonship by God, but also to Melchizedek, king of Salem and eternal priest of the most high God.

The legendary Apostle Paulos or Paul, author of the earliest-known Christian texts, invokes *both* figures when he quotes King David's Psalms 2 and 110 in Hebrews 5, *"So also Christ did not glorify Himself so as to become a high priest, but He [God] who said to Him, 'You are my son, today I have begotten you,' just as He [God] says also in another passage, 'You are a priest forever according to the order of Melchizedek.'"* Paul goes on to describe Melchizedek as *"Without father, without mother, without descent, having neither beginning of days, nor end of life; but made like unto the Son of God; abideth a priest continually"* (Hebrews 7:3).

Paul emphasizes that King David's Psalms are crucial to Yahushwa's own message that God offers you the same unconditional love and filial adoption originally offered to David, and that you potentially hold Melchizedek's eternal and transcendental priesthood outside of space-time: a beautiful description of the Wholeness from which you unconditionally love and minister to your wavicles.

Life of Yahushwa as a Model of Wavicle Work

The various milestones of Yahushwa's life beautifully map the Initiations or states of consciousness your wavicles (and you) may encounter in Wavicle Work:

His *birth* represents the birth of the Witness, wherein you witness the wavicle as a separate being inside your body, and in turn may experience being witnessed by your own Wholeness.

His *baptism* is the milestone of celestial consciousness, when you appear to your wavicle as its parent or personal God, telling it, *"You are my child in whom my soul delights; whatever you most need is yours!"* while flooding it with unconditional love and support. In turn you yourself may experience the currents of unconditional love and support from your own Wholeness.

His *transfiguration* on the mountain, when his face *"did shine as the sun"* as he spoke with Moses and Elias and a voice out of the cloud called him *"my beloved Son,"* corresponds to enlightenment or unity, when your wavicle responds to your love and whole-heartedly aligns and harmonizes with the light of your awareness. In turn you may experience the grace of enlightenment, attaining the subjective omnipresence of light-speed.

His *crucifixion and resurrection* represent the realization of your wavicle that it is no longer a separate wavicle but is indeed nothing or no-thing, the *empty* part of the emptiful Wholeness. The crucifixion is literally the *crossing* and merging of Spirit and Matter across what had been the separate wavicle or intermediary Soul. In turn you may cross the Void, beginning subjectively to move faster than light and backwards in time.

His *ascension* represents your wavicle's identification with you as the paradoxical Wholeness of everything, the *full* part of the emptiful Wholeness, containing an infinity of wavicles: As John (12:32) quotes Yahushwa, *"If I be lifted up from the earth, I will draw all men unto me."* In turn you may experience the reality of your own ascension, mastery and ministry to your countless lost "past-selves" or wavicles, drawing them into eternal Wholeness.

Reconciliation and the Golden Rule

Yahushwa was most certainly a Master of Wavicle Work. Over and over again he describes the process of aligning wholeheartedly with Wholeness or God, and turning within, finding the "outer" pain within yourself, and loving your wavicles or little children as if they are your angels, co-creating your kingdom of heaven through reconciliation and the Golden Rule:

"You shall love the Lord your God with all your heart and soul and strength. This is the great and foremost commandment. And the second is like it: you shall love your neighbor as yourself. On these two commandments depend the whole Law and the Prophets." First, align yourself completely with Wholeness, then communicate the unconditional love of that Wholeness to everyone as yourself. Everyone in your environment is a reflection or projection of one of your wavicles. By remembering

this, you can re-member them, love them, integrate them, and convert them from "demonic" to "divine."

"Don't resist evil." That which you resist persists, as something not-Self, not-God, and remains within your awareness field as a knot of rejection and suffering: a morsel of spiritual indigestion and "heartburn." You can resolve evil via wavicle work: wholeheartedly allowing it to *be*; as you begin to realize it is a portion of your Wholeness, it also becomes a portion of Holiness. Love flows into it and enlightens it into the bliss of release. Pain is never caused by the particular flavor of the wavicle of God you are rejecting; it is always your very act of rejection or resisting the wavicle which causes you pain, as you are at that moment believing in the lie of duality. By making something not-divine, you give it the power to overshadow the divine.

"The Kingdom of God is within you." "Seek first the kingdom of Heaven, and all else will be added unto you." Your deep fulfillment never truly resides in your environment; it lies within you as the finest feeling level. As you establish that inner contentment it radiates into your environment which then reflects your feeling level. The wavicles are your senses; by clarifying and integrating them, you clarify and integrate the environment they perceive or create.

"Judge not, lest ye be judged." Whenever you judge someone or something, you separate yourself from it as if that wavicle is not really your own expression. When you judge a wavicle you are telling the universe you don't understand it, and you will then automatically be moved to act as that wavicle yourself, so you will understand it from the inside. When you cut a wavicle off from you, you yourself will quickly feel cut off and alienated. Whatever energy you devote to your wavicles, you very quickly experience yourself, as a feedback loop to encourage you to attune to and emanate your highest and deepest essence of unconditional Love, Light, and Laughter.

"Take the log out of your own eye before attending to the speck in your neighbor's eye." Do wavicle work to change your environment; it is much easier and more effective to comb your own

hair and watch your reflection change, than it is to try to comb the mirror.

"Allow the little children to come to Me, and do not hinder them, for of such is the kingdom of Heaven." Allow your wavicles, your thought-children, to come home to you, the unconditionally loving "I AM"; when you acknowledge their innate divinity, you re-enter Heaven, for these wavicles are your own senses.

"Unless you are converted, and become like little children, you shall not enter the kingdom of Heaven." "What you do to the smallest of these, you do to Me." As you practice wavicle work, you allow your thought-children to remember they are divine. You enter into your own creation by collapsing and converting or turning inward into your own wavicles or senses, thereby vividly experiencing the effects of your own thoughts. When you bless your wavicle-children, you become blessed; as you bring them Home, you re-enter Heaven.

You actually serve your own wavicles as their Christ, their emissary of the Father's unconditional Love and Light and Laughter. You bring them salvation from suffering, as you call them out of ignorance to rejoice in harmony as the divinely awakened members of your *Ecclesia*, your church, your body – the body of Christ. Your body of wavicles or devatas is your Mother Divine, the Mother-Nature of God, your Sacred Matter, your *Ecclesia Mater* or Mother Church, your creation.

Christianity and the Hermetic Tradition

Following the teachings of St. Paul, early Christianity reflected the Hermetic view of humans as a trinity of Body, Soul, and Spirit. From the fourth century CE, however, the church began to favor St. Augustine's model of a simple dichotomy of Body and Soul. As the relationship of humanity to Spirit became wholly "other," the understanding of humans as a microcosm of Wholeness was lost. Theurgy, the "divine work" of uniting with God through perfecting one's own consciousness, gave way to dependence upon grace dispensed through the ecclesiastical hierarchy. Though the church retained St. Paul's idea of *theosis* or union with God through filial adoption, the unity became one of love, not of substance.

The rediscovery of the Hermetic texts by the West in 1460 sparked the Italian Renaissance and inspired many Christian scholars like Marisilio Ficino, Giordano Bruno, and Pico della Mirandola with visions of the *prisca theologia*, the original theology given by God to humanity imparting the truth of the trinity of Spirit, Soul, and Body. They believed all religions yet retained the "original theology" in more or less diluted form.

The surfacing in 1945 of the ancient scriptures in the Nag Hammadi Library, including the *Gospel of Thomas*, *Gospel of Philip*, *Gospel of Truth*, and *The Thunder: Perfect Mind*, clarified the controversial roles that Gnosticism and Hermeticism played in the rise of early Christianity. Elaine Pagels (*The Gnostic Paul: Gnostic Exegesis of the Pauline Letters)* has shown that Valentinus (c. 100-160 CE) and his Gnostic Christians claimed their spiritual descent directly from the Apostle Paul himself via his secret teachings to Theudas.

After rejecting their Gnostic and Hermetic currents in favor of the Roman-era literal, historical Jesus, "Orthodox" Christians generally echoed Judaism's distrust of astrology, and perhaps with good cause, as used improperly it can breed fatalism. However, many scholars have affirmed a subtle *astrotheology* in Christianity, citing solar attributes in Yahushwa, the golden-haloed "Sun of Righteousness," with his 12 disciples as the 12 months of the solar year, with Christmas celebrating the sun's "rebirth" after the dark midwinter solstice, and with Easter celebrating the sun's crossing or "crucifixion" into the light half of the year after the midspring equinox.

The archetypal cross itself appears in the "fixed cross" of the zodiac, denoted by the "four beasts" of the Evangelists: the Lion of Leo, the Eagle of Scorpio, the Man of Aquarius, and the Ox of Taurus, derived from the same four "living creatures" of Ezekiel 1:10. Followers of Yahushwa identified themselves with the Fish symbol not only because the acronym ICHTHYS ("fish" in Greek) stands for Iesous Christos, Theou Yios, Soter ("Jesus Christ, God's Son, Savior"), but also to commemorate his spiritual inauguration of the Age of Pisces, the Fish.

While eschewing alchemy as a rule, orthodox Christianity maintains a beautiful Alchemical Mystery as the centerpiece of its Mass, wherein ordinary bread and wine are transubstantiated into the radiant "body and blood" of God and thence taken into one's own body at communion, potentially refining your perception of your entire creation into celestial gold. Likewise, blessing all of your food can alchemically transmute it and your body into the living presence of Wholeness and Holiness.

Some Christian exemplars of Wavicle Work

Some of the many inspiring Christian "patron saints" of Wavicle Work include the Essenes, Paul, Valentinus, Origen, Clement of Alexandria, Bernard of Clairvaux, Francis of Assisi, Meister Eckhart, Julian of Norwich, John of the Cross, Marsilio Ficino, Giordano Bruno, Jacob Boehme, John Donne, and the mysterious translator of the King James Bible: perhaps an exiled Edward de Vere, 17th Earl of Oxford, who many believe was the master-poet better known as William Shake-Spear.

Wavicle Work in Islam

Islam and Reconciliation

The word *Islam* has been translated as "surrender," meaning a surrender of your separate will to the will of God. This is the essence of Particle Prayer, wherein you long for and attune yourself as creature to your Creator, who is "nearer to a man than his jugular vein." And it is the essence of Wavicle Work, wherein you convey the message of the unconditional love of God the Creator, the all-merciful, the all-compassionate, to the separate creatures within your *Ummah* or "body of believers." The call to surrender to unconditional love is a call to Spirit-

Matter reconciliation. Surrendering to divine perfection completely unites heavenly Spirit and earthly Matter.

Some Islamic exemplars of the Hermetic Tradition and Wavicle Work

The young Muhammad accompanied his uncle's trading caravans to Egypt, Yemen, Syria, and Mesopotamia, where he spoke with the various holy men he met. Islam sees itself as a reformation or revival of the ancient religion of Abraham, of which Judaism and Christianity are also branches. Muhammad traced his descent from Ishmael, son of Abraham and of the Pharaoh's royal handmaiden, Hagar. As noted above, it seems likely that Abraham was a contemporary and brother-in-law of Pharaoh Tahut-moses III, who we believe was later known variously as King David, Melchizedek, and Hermes Trismegistus, and is an original "patron saint" of Wavicle Work. Islam recognizes King David or Dawud as a prophet, messenger, lawgiver of God, and righteous king. Muslim scholars equate Hermes Trismegistus with Idris, a prophet the Qur'an calls "trustworthy and patient" and "exalted to a high station."

While Christian Europe was deep in the Dark Ages, Islam enjoyed a Golden Age of scholarship and discovery, having carefully preserved ancient wisdom long lost to the West. The Ismaili and other Shi'ite sects of Islam were particularly steeped in Hermeticism and Neoplatonism. The eighth-century Iranian genius Abu Musa Jabir ibn Hayyan (Latinized as "Geber") excelled in alchemy, astrology, medicine, engineering, and geography, inspired by Hermes Trismegistus as well as the Greeks, the Neoplatonist Porphyry, the Egyptian alchemists Zosimos and Agathodaimon, and others. The many alchemical works attributed to Jabir ibn Hayyan constituted an Ismaili corpus of scriptures dedicated to making the elixir of perfect balance between the hidden and the manifest: the Wavicle Work of aligning your Soul (your creature or wavicle) to mediate between your transcendental Spirit (your Creator) and your manifest Body (your creation).

Jabir himself was called "the Sufi," and the mystical heart of Islam is that *gnosis* or transcendental heart-knowledge of God known as Sufism, also derived largely from the Hermetic doctrines of Ancient Egypt. Among Jabir's many works, the *Second Book of the Elements of Foundation* contained a translation of the Emerald Tablet of Hermes Trismegistus, following the earlier *Book of the Secret of Creation and the Art of Nature*, attributed to "Balinas" or Apollonius of Tyana.

Another important early Sufi master was the alchemist and thaumaturge Dhul-Nun al-Misri ("the Egyptian") (796-859), who reportedly gained his wisdom from his clairvoyant reading of Ancient Egyptian hieroglyphs. Other early Sufi masters like Ibn Sina (Latinized as Avicenna) (980-1037), Shahab ad-Din Yahya ibn Habash as-Suhrawardi (1155-1191), and the great 'Abu 'Abdillah Muhammad ibn 'Ali ibn Muhammad ibn 'Arabi (known as ibn 'Arabi) (1165-1240) also traced their wisdom back to the Wavicle Work of Hermes Trismegistus and Ancient Egypt.

Perhaps the most famous Sufi in the West is the immensely popular Persian mystical poet, Jalal ad-Din Muhammad Rumi (1207-1273). He is one of the world's best exponents of Wavicle Work:

You personify God's message.
You reflect the King's face.
There is nothing in the universe that you are not.
Everything you want, look for it within yourself—
You are that.

And again,

They are the chosen ones
Who have surrendered.
Once they were particles of light
Now they are the radiant sun.

How beautiful is Rumi's heartfelt description of your wavicles' reconciliation and homecoming!

Islam and the Golden Rule

Islam clearly expresses the Golden Rule in several places: In Kirab al-Kafi, vol. 2, p. 146, Muhammad says simply, *"As you would have people do to you, do to them; and what you dislike to be done to you, don't do to them."* In An-Nawawi's Forty Hadith 13, Muhammad says, *"None of you will believe until you wish for your brother what you wish for yourself,"* or *"...love your brother as you love yourself."* And in Surah 24, the Quran says, *"... and you should forgive And overlook: Do you not like God to forgive you? And Allah is The Merciful Forgiving."*

Wavicle Work in Taoism (Daoism)

Taoism and Reconciliation

Developed by the legendary Chinese sages Lao-tzu (Lao-Tze, Laozi) (c. 6th century BCE) and Chuang-tzu (Zhuang Zhou, Zhuangzi) (c. 4th century BCE), Taoism advocates *Wu Wei*, meaning "non-doing" or "non-effort" by trusting, surrendering into, and becoming one with the *Tao*, the 'eternally nameless' and indefinable yet fundamentally knowable nature of the Universe. This is precisely what Wavicle Work uncovers: That we have ever rested in and as the Tao or Wholeness, and that all doing is actually done by our wavicles automatically, in obedience to our conscious or unconscious programming. How we treat them is how Wholeness treats us, and as we continue to bring our wavicles home into us, through them we in turn continue to enter and re-enter the Tao.

The Tao consists of a constant interplay and perfect balance of complementary and interdependent opposites: the so-called "masculine," bright, solar, active, contracted, heavenly, or *Yang* energies, and the so-called "feminine," dark, lunar, passive, expanded, earthly, or *Yin* energies. These are what we have called Spirit or Creator, and Matter or Creation. In Wavicle Work you can often relieve a specific wavicle by offering it such opposites: e.g., "I give you infinitely divine rest (*Yin*) and infinitely divine activity (*Yang*) simultaneously, now and forever!" to bring it back into us, or the ineffable Wholeness, or the Tao.

Taoism and Hermeticism

As in Hermeticism, Taoism maintains an interest in both Astrology and Alchemy. Taoist Astrology is similar to the Hermetic Astrology of the West in that it divides the zodiacal circle into twelve equal sections governed by animals, but each animal rules for a year within a twelve-year cycle (an orbit of Jupiter), rather than Western astrology's month within an annual cycle (an apparent orbit of the sun).

Taoist astrologers also apply a system of five elements or phases via the flow-patterns of a pentagram in a manner foreign to modern western astrology but reminiscent of Hermetic magic and of Pythagoras, who adopted the pentagram as the symbol of his school and applied five elements to it, reportedly gaining his knowledge of geometry from the Egyptians. As noted in the section on Wicca, advanced Wavicle Work archetypal studies show a pattern of four interlocking pentacles around the Solar Calendar year, with one point of each pentagram opening to an equinox or solstice and the other four points in signs of each of the four elements.

Internal Taoist Alchemy promotes cultivation of the Three Treasures of Vital Bodily Essence (*Ching* or *Jing*), Spirit or Breath (*Chi* or *Qi*), and Soul, Mind, or Radiant Consciousness (*Shen*) – the same Trinity of Body, Spirit and Soul we have seen since Ancient Egypt and which are employed in Wavicle Work – to attain the Golden Elixir, described like the Hermetic Philosopher's Stone as a red-gold source of immortality.

Taoism and the Golden Rule

The *Tao Te Ching* (chapter 49) says, *"The sage has no interest of his own, but takes the interest of the people as his own. He is kind to the kind; he is also kind to the unkind: for Virtue is kind. He is faithful to the faithful; he is also faithful to the unfaithful: for Virtue is faithful."*

94

Li Ying Chang's *Tai Shang Ying Pian*, or *Lao Tse's Treatise on the Response of the Tao*, says, *"Regard your neighbor's gain as your own gain, and your neighbor's loss as your own loss."* Both of these are excellent descriptions of the practice of Wavicle Work, for your neighbor is essentially your own wavicle.

Wavicle Work in Hinduism

Krishna and Wavicle Work

Hindus revere Krishna as an avatar or divine incarnation of the great god Vishnu, whom we would call the embodiment of Love. A devotee who has fully harmonized with Krishna and his *shakti*-goddess Radha (sometimes considered an avatar of Lakshmi), in Krishna-Consciousness perceives *Goloka Vrindavan*, the supreme yet sensually celestial realm of Krishna's own creation, wherein every being is both a spark of one's own "I AM" consciousness and also one's devotee. This is a beautiful description of the potential results of Wavicle Work, wherein you lovingly align your wavicles, devatas, or devotees with your Self as Wholeness, creating countless "bubble-worlds" for your devotees to enjoy, or in Particle Prayer align yourself as devotee with your Creator, and either way in so doing enjoy the devata's sensory fulfilment of Heaven on Earth.

Shiva, Alchemy, and Wavicle Work

In addition to Vishnu and his avatars, Hindus also revere the great god Shiva and his *shakti* Parvati, whom we would call the embodiments of Bliss. The Hindu scriptures contain a marvelous account of Wavicle Work in their myth of Rudra or Shiva and the asuras, or demons. As the demons are Shiva's children, they do *tapas* or penance for many thousands of years, suffering austerities in order to gain their divine father's attention. And when they do, he invariably offers them a boon: whatever they most desire. Similarly, when you practice Wavicle Work you can play the role of Shiva, attending to the painful suffering of your wavicles by offering them unconditional Love as your own children, welcoming them home and giving them whatever they most desire.

Shiva traditionally unfolds the secrets of alchemy, and Wavicle Work alchemically transforms your demons from leaden nuggets of resistance back into your golden devatas or devotees, enlightening them – and you – through unconditional Love into the immortal bliss of the eternal Now. The paradoxical nature of the Now is like liquid mercury; it is infinitely reflective and impossible for the dualistic intellect to pin down or grasp. Mercury is considered to be Shiva's seed, and the Hindu word for alchemy is *rasasiddhi*, meaning "perfection attained by means of quicksilver." This mercury is the universal mercury, also known as Azoth: the Universal Solvent, the Life within All, the Original Self.

Reconciliation of Spirit and Matter

Like Ancient Egypt, India acknowledges a Trinity of Spirit, Body, and Soul. Spirit is the Hindus' *Rishi*, the Seer, your subjective pure awareness; the Body is *Chhandas*, the Meter or Measurable: the Seen, your material objective world; and the Soul is *Devata*, the Seeing, your process which reconciles the two. These again are the Creator (Rishi), the Creation (Chhandas), and the intermediary Creature (Devata) through which the Creator senses and enjoys Creation, awareness of which is enlivened in Wavicle Work.

Hindus also divide Reality into a trinity of eternal qualities or *gunas* which they call *Sat* (Being), *Chit* (Consciousness), and *Ananda* (Bliss). These three eternal gunas are reflected into space-time creation as *Sat* becomes *Sattva* or centripetal coherence, *Chit* becomes *Rajas* or rotational activity, and *Ananda* becomes *Tamas* or centrifugal dissolution. (This is True *Tamas*, not the false *tamas* of ignorance caused by a refusal to accept a wavicle in *Sat*.)

The gunas are personalized as the Hindu *Trimurti* or Divine Trinity of Brahma the Golden Creator, Indra or Vishnu the Blue

Maintainer, and Rudra or Shiva the Red Destroyer. Each of these gods has his own feminine counterpart or *shakti*: Brahma has Saraswati; Vishnu has Lakshmi, and Shiva has Parvati, or Mata Devi. Hindus ascribe the sacred *AUM* to the Trinity, usually giving *A* to Brahma, *U* to Vishnu, and *M* to Shiva. The whole of *AUM* is contained in seed-form within the first letter, "*A.*"

The path of Reconciliation is called *Yoga*, or "Union." In his famed Yoga Sutras, the great sage Patanjali outlined the eight branches of *Raja* ("Royal") or *Ashtanga* ("eight-limbed") Yoga: 1) *yamas* or ethical self-restraints (including non-violence, non-coveting, truthfulness, non-stealing, and chastity), 2) *niyamas* or virtues (including purity, contentment, *tapas* to focus desire through suffering austerities, introspection, and surrender into Wholeness), 3) *asanas* or physical postures, 4) *pranayama* or breath-control, 5) *pratyahara* or withdrawal of the senses, 6) *dharana* or mental concentration, 7) *dhyana* or meditation, and 8) *samadhi* or ecstatic transcendence.

Wavicle Work generally embraces limbs 1) and 2) through connecting with your Creator-Self, both formless (beyond violence, coveting, lying, stealing, and lust) and containing all perfect qualities (including purity and contentment), and thus satisfying all of your wavicle-self's needs on the subtlest-feeling level (loving your wavicle's tapasic suffering through self-awareness into ecstatic surrender). Wavicle Work specifically embraces limbs 3), 4), and 5) through attending to your body (*asana*), letting it breathe (*pranayama*), and localizing your wavicle (*pratyahara*); and limbs 6), 7), and 8) through communing with your wavicle in the naturally-unfolding process of attentive Love (*dharana*), conscious Light (*dhyana*), and blissful Laughter (*samadhi*).

Besides Raja Yoga, there are many other traditional Yogic paths to suit the needs and predilections of seekers at any given time. These include *Hatha* Yoga for the physical body, *Kundalini* or *Laya* Yoga for the subtle-energy body, *Karma* Yoga for daily selfless work, *Bhakti* Yoga for devotion to God, and *Jnana* Yoga for intellectual understanding and pure knowledge of the Self as the paradoxical *Brahman*. From the legendary Veda Vyasa to Adi Shankara (c. 700-750 CE) to now, an unbroken lineage of Hindu sages have taught *Vedanta*, the "end of the Vedas," reconciling Spirit and Matter in *Advaita* or nondualism as the realization of Brahman, the Self as the emptiful Wholeness, both *nirguna* and *saguna*: nothing and everything. Vedanta shines forth eternally in the four principal *Mahavakyas* or Great Sayings: *"I am That; Thou art That; All this is That; That alone is."*

You can give your wavicles and thus experience for yourself all of the benefits of any of these Yogas, including the understanding and experience of Brahman, by bringing them home into you, the container of all possibilities and all opposites.

Some nondualist *advaitins* deny the reality or importance of Matter, seeing it as only a dream or "story" unworthy of attention. Wavicle Work demonstrates that Matter is as much a part of Wholeness as Spirit. Perhaps the most profound reconciliation of Spirit and Matter in Hinduism is in *Tantra*, which arose in the early centuries of the Common Era and affirms the utter reality and divinity of both aspects. Though Tantra has been concretized into "sacred sexuality" in the West, it traditionally celebrates the practitioner's full reconciliation and alchemical marriage of God and Goddess, Spirit and Matter, on all levels. Tantra's whole-hearted embrace of all of life is precisely the approach of Wavicle Work.

Hinduism and the Golden Rule

In the great epic *Mahabharata*, the wise Vidura advises King Yudhisthira: *"All worlds are balanced on dharma; dharma encompasses ways to prosperity as well. O King, dharma is the best quality to have, wealth the medium and desire the lowest. Hence (keeping these in mind), by self-control and by making dharma your main focus, treat others as you treat yourself."* While we feel dharma, prosperity, desire, and liberation are all equally valid goals in Wavicle Work, Vidura's final six-word summation of the Golden Rule – *treat others as you treat yourself* – is both succinct and beautiful.

Wavicle Work in Buddhism

Buddhism and Reconciliation

Siddhartha Gautama Buddha (c. 623-543 BCE), the founder of Buddhism, reportedly said, "I have taught one thing and one thing only: suffering (*dukkha*) and the cessation of suffering." This is also Wavicle Work's main teaching.

The Buddha taught in part as a reaction to the Hinduism of his time. While he acknowledged the existence of the Vedic gods, he denied that they were superior to human beings and rejected the Brahmin priests' hierarchical caste system and rituals for placating the gods. In placing the ability and responsibility for cessation of suffering squarely within the consciousness of the suffering individual, the Buddha revived the Ancient Mysteries and expressed the fundamental principles of Wavicle Work.

When you practice Wavicle Work, you "worship" or "show the worth of" your various devatas or divine wavicles from the standpoint of their creator, consciousness itself; when you practice Particle Prayer, you are acknowledging your Creator as your own larger self or source. In either form of Wavicle Work, you are remembering your original nature beyond your separate self, and establishing a dialogue between you as creature and you as Creator.

Buddhists believe that the infinite span of time has seen not merely one, but many Buddhas: human beings who have realized the impermanence of the self, through *Nirvana* or "blowing out" of the separate ego. The Wavicle Work system shows that when a wavicle experiences Nirvana, Spirit and Matter meet and merge in the sacred heart or solar plexus, eclipsing the Ahamkara or separate "I AM" Soul there in the Awakening or Realization of the emptiful Void or paradoxical Wholeness. The Wholeness expands to unite the *Manasic* realm of the animalistic lower mind in the navel with the *Buddhic* realm of the finest-feeling level of intuition in the heart.

Your awakened heart contains two polarities: the *receiving* side of Enlightened Prosperity, which we could call *Siddhartha* or perfect earth-mastery, perfect abundance; and the *giving* side of Loving Justice or Compassionate Right Action, which we could call *Sattvadharma*. All of these titles have been applied to realizers of the Buddha-nature: *Siddhartha Buddha*; *Bodhisattva*, *Bodhidharma*.

The emptiful Void or Wholeness, your own Buddha-nature, contains an infinite number of wavicles, or devatas. One of the duties of the Awakened One, the Buddha, is to teach and enlighten the devas or devatas. As you identify your wavicles or devatas and pay attention to them in unconditional love, letting them simply *be* as a fundamental part of your Wholeness, you naturally enlighten them. Non-labelling attention *is* unconditional love. By paying full attention only to the localized story or issue, your unconditional love transforms it from pain through light into bliss. Pain and pleasure are born of duality-stories, but bliss really is not; it is one of the primordial expressions of Wholeness.

Buddhist monks allegedly taught a technique of breath and non-dual attention to resolve even the most intense bodily pain into bliss. Assuredly it may take considerable practice to discover and maintain the requisite clarity of mind and laser-like focus of attention. If the mind even begins to slip off this present moment-place of sensation, the pain may reappear. However, even a little of this practice may accomplish considerable healing.

Of the three traditional forms of Buddhism, *Theravada* is the oldest and most "orthodox." Practiced mostly by monks, it is the path of the *Arhat*, one who attains personal liberation from rebirth. This describes the initial steps of Wavicle Work, where you remember that you are not your wavicles. By localizing your predominant wavicle, you remember that you are not your story; you are not bound by time and space. In essence, you have always been liberated.

The second form of Buddhism is *Mahayana*, the path of the *Bodhisattva*, the spiritual practitioner who delays his or her own complete liberation to seek enlightenment for all sentient beings first. While this has been called the "Bodhisattva vow," it appears like the "Bodhisattva predicament:" not really a decision so much as a realization. It equates to the latter steps of Wavicle Work, wherein you realize that whatever you do for your wavicles, you do for yourself. Even though you as Wholeness are fundamentally detached and non-localized, if your localized wavicles are suffering in ignorance – and everyone in your body of awareness is your wavicle – then in a sense, so are you. Your ultimate happiness and enlightenment depends upon theirs, as they are in you and you are in them.

Mahayana Buddhists acknowledge a kind of Trinity in their doctrine of *Trikaya*, or three bodies of a Buddha: First, the *Dharmakaya* or *Truth body* of boundless and infinite enlightenment; second, the *Sambhogakaya* or *mutual-enjoyment body* of luminous clear light; and third, the *Nirmanakaya* or *created body* appearing in space-time. These appear to equate to the Ancient Egyptian and Hermetic divisions of Spirit, Soul, and Body: particularly as the Dharmakaya Samantabhadra (and his equivalent, Vajradhara) is dark blue in color like the Egyptian Amen and Hindu Vishnu/Krishna.

One of the most profound methods of Spirit-Matter reconciliation has been meditation. The fifth-century Persian or Indian monk Bodhidharma transmitted the Mahayana Buddhist techniques of meditation (Sanskrit *Dhyan*) into China where they were called *Chan,* and passing later into Japan they became known as *Zen.* Wavicle Work effects a similar communication and reconciliation between these three bodies by conveying the highest spiritual Truth of the *Dharmakayic* unconditional love and compassion through your *Sambhogakayic* conscious soul or wavicle-mind and thence into your *Nirmanakayic* body of space-time.

The third form of Buddhism is *Vajrayana* or Tantric, which probably contains the clearest expression of the principles of Wavicle Work. In the eleventh century, the great Tibetan Buddhist yogini Machig Labdron unfolded the Vajrayana Buddhist *chod* technique of nourishing one's mental demons to convert them to allies, as beautifully described in Lama Tsultrim Allione's *Feeding Your Demons: Ancient Wisdom for Resolving Inner Conflict*. This feeding-not-fighting tactic is precisely the same integrative approach of reconciliation you use in Wavicle Work.

Buddhism and the Golden Rule

In *Sutta Nipata* 705, Buddha says, *"Comparing oneself to others in such terms as 'Just as I am so are they; just as they are so am I,"* he should neither kill nor cause others to kill."* In Dhammapada 10 he says, *"One who, while himself seeking happiness, oppresses with violence other beings who also desire happiness, will not attain happiness hereafter."* Though in the negative "Silver Rule" form, as "Do not do unto others what you would not have them do unto you," these clearly express the reciprocal spirit of Wavicle Work's Golden Rule, wherein it becomes self-evident that you are treating yourself exactly how you are treating "others" in your awareness: your own wavicles.

Chapter Eight

Psychotherapy and Wavicle Work

Psychotherapy provides the fundamental insight that a suppressed or repressed issue must be brought fully into consciousness for it to be healed. This is the natural process and result of Wavicle Work, which provides a swift, effortless technique to meet the "frozen" wavicle in unconditional love where it is, bring it into the full light of awareness, and meet its needs unreservedly in the context of Wholeness.

Wavicle Work is intended to help those who are already relatively happy and well-adjusted to reach their ultimate goals of passion, prosperity, right action, and liberation. It has not been tested extensively on those with pronounced psychiatric illness or disorders, and is not recommended as a substitute for any conventional psychotherapies or healing modalities. That said, people encountering Wavicle Work are sometimes tempted to compare and contrast it to various psychotherapeutic growth techniques. This chapter briefly looks at some of the similarities and differences between them and Wavicle Work. I have arranged the techniques by their approximate dates of development.

Freud, Jung, Adler, and Wavicle Work

The three luminaries of modern psychoanalysis and depth psychology, pioneers of the unconscious mind, were Sigmund Freud, Carl G. Jung, and Alfred Adler. Wavicle Work owes something to each of them.

Sigmund Freud

Sigmund Freud (1856-1939) founded psychoanalysis, exploring the unconscious minds of his patients with techniques like free-association and dream analysis. Freud divided the personality or psyche into *id, ego, and superego*, to a degree anticipating our tripartite model of *Manasic* ("animal" mental), *Ahamkara* ("I AM" causal), and *Buddhic* ("ancestral" intuitive) soul, located in the navel, solar-plexus, and heart, respectively. Countering the prudishness of his strait-laced age, Freud traced nearly everything back to the id's sexuality and libido, which we would call *the passion and liberation in the loins* or sex chakra, and to the id's aggressive death-urge, which we would call *the passion and liberation in the belly* or navel chakra.

Freud also discovered the Oedipus complex and concomitant castration anxiety, wherein a young child unconsciously desires to mate with its opposite-sex parent, and consequently fears genital mutilation by its "rival" same-sex parent. The complex is named for the mythical Greek king who accidentally slew his father and married his mother. Advanced Wavicle-Work calendar studies show all the planetary Archetypes witnessing the seasonal "death" of their same-sex parent, and two of the Archetypes "die" seasonally by sexual mutilation. However, the Archetypes do not marry their parents but their siblings, as in Egyptian theology and royalty. Interestingly, Freud was also the first modern thinker to connect Moses and Akhenaton, as described in his last book, *Moses and Monotheism* (1939).

A friend had studied Freud in school but his spiritual path eschewed psychoanalysis, and Freud's insights had never seemed relevant until about three and one half years after discovering Wavicle Work. Noticing a repeating pattern of infidelity across several relationships, he then looked inside, past the "poor me" victim-program, to see who was actually creating this drama of intense jealousy, rage, and suffering, and was shocked to discover the Oedipus Complex in one of his own wavicles, a three-year-old self. He was repeatedly manifesting another male to play the part of his father, with whom he could then compete for his mother, played sequentially by his partners.

About six months later, acutely painful memories of psychic castration also surfaced from the same time-period, albeit self-inflicted as a rejection of violent paternal energies. Fortunately, some Wavicle Work first gave his child-self his ideal Mother-Goddess and then healed this deep psychic wound permanently, giving him a new-found appreciation of the genius of Sigmund Freud.

C. G. Jung

Carl Gustav Jung (1865-1961) left Freud's circle in 1914 and focused on the profoundly powerful realm of *Archetypes*, eternal and universal figures like the Great Mother and Father, the Child, the Devil, the Wise Old Man and Woman, the Trickster, and the Hero: many of which appear in advanced Wavicle Work. Jung discovered that the Archetypes emerged from the *Collective Unconscious*, the realm of the *Pleroma*: a Gnostic term meaning *fullness*, but which Jung defined as a "Nothingness … both empty and full." He also developed the concepts of synchronicity, the complex, the shadow, extraversion vs. introversion, the anima and animus, the self, individuation, and the theories of personality behind the Meyers-Briggs personality test. Perhaps most importantly, Jung was in every sense a Hermeticist: an intrepid explorer of the soul-realms of astrology, alchemy, and theurgy, the "divine work" of uniting with God or Wholeness. Unlike Freud, he felt that spiritual experience of the numinous was necessary for human health.

In our system the Pleroma or fullness of the archetypal realm dwells in your third-eye chakra as a meeting of the *lunar liberation* and *solar passion*, which we would agree with Jung in calling the *coniunctio*, the Marriage of the Sun and Moon. But the emptiful Void or paradoxical Wholeness which Jung also calls the Pleroma, is for us more than the Pleroma's traditional fullness: In the emptiful Wholeness, Spirit descends and Matter ascends to meet and mingle as the Ineffable in your sacred heart, expanding from there to embrace your whole body of awareness. Nonetheless in his intrepid exploration of archetypes, integration of the shadow, and dedicated Hermeticism, Jung is truly a "patron saint" of Wavicle Work.

Alfred Adler

Alfred Adler (1870-1937) split from Freud's circle in 1911 and founded *individual psychology*, emphasizing the person as an indivisible whole. He discovered the inferiority complex and emphasized both the holism of the individual and his connection with the social world. He acknowledged the individual's need for power and cooperation in order to accomplish specific life-tasks: love and sexuality, occupation and work, and society and friendship.

Adler delved deeper than Freud had done into what advanced Wavicle Work would call the navel chakra's "animal mind" and its issues of fight-or-flight and power. Also in acknowledging the connection of the whole individual with his world, Adler anticipated the larger understanding of basic Wavicle Work, wherein an individual *and* his or her creation or reality are appreciated as essentially one holistic entity.

TM, the TM-Sidhi Program, and Wavicle Work

Among the many modern proponents of self-help and enlightenment, one of the most famous has been Maharishi Mahesh Yogi (1918-2008). Developed from the early 1950s through the 1970s, his Transcendental Meditation (TM) and TM-Sidhi Programs are expressly designed to bring the meditator into spiritual and material fulfillment through the enlightening experience of seven states of consciousness – not only deep sleep, dream, and waking, but also transcendence, Cosmic Consciousness, God Consciousness, and Unity Consciousness. The TM-Sidhi program integrates both *asanas* or physical yoga postures and *pranayama* or breathing techniques to your meditation along with specific *siddhis* or "perfections" from Patanjali's Yoga Sutras to enliven all the possibilities inherent in the finest-feeling level from which your reality emerges. Though individual results certainly vary, I found my nine-year practice of these programs to deliver virtually everything promised.

At your core, however, you are not really in space-time; as Wholeness or "Brahman" itself you are both *nirguna* and *saguna*, nothing and everything, the ultimate container of space-time. And so you yourself are not actually evolving through various states of consciousness: but your wavicles are, and you experience these states through your wavicles. Wavicle Work naturally enlivens the appreciation of these additional states of consciousness.

When you first pay attention to an internal wavicle, you lose yourself in it, thinking you are that wavicle. This is where you always begin the work: from ignorance, identifying with the thought. You then can transcend your identification with your wavicle by withdrawing your senses inward from the projected reality, localizing them in a tension-point in your body and becoming its witness, thereby giving that wavicle Cosmic Consciousness. You then put your thought-wavicle in God Consciousness by acting as its Creator, offering it unconditional love, and giving it whatever it most desires. And you give it Unity Consciousness by reminding it of its inherent divinity and allowing it to merge with you, completely aligning with the light of your awareness if it so desires. And you can introduce it to Brahman, the crystallinely mercurial, paradoxical self itself, by presenting your wavicle with simultaneously opposite ideas, thus bringing it completely out of duality.

Whatever you give your wavicles you experience, and even though you are inherently beyond space and time and thereby beyond permanent identification with any specific states of consciousness, you will simultaneously enjoy whatever you give your wavicles, including evolution and enlightenment.

Wavicle Work can be seen as a kind of personalized sutra program, where you give your wavicles whatever they most need in this moment on the finest feeling level. From here their perfect ("siddhi") fulfilment quickly and naturally flows into all of creation in the most harmonious and life-supporting manner. You are not in charge of *how* your wavicles manifest your desires; you are only in charge of giving them the OK to do so in the most harmonious and natural way, through establishing that finest feeling level of fulfillment.

Focusing and Wavicle Work

Created by psychotherapists Eugene Gendlin and Carl Rogers in the 1950s and 1960s after years of studying successful psycho-therapeutic interactions, Focusing trains you to refer to your "felt sense" or bodily awareness in order to go beneath your intellect to enliven a holistic, *a priori* experience of the world. This bodily awareness is itself is a great relief and a genuine form of liberation. I have not practiced Focusing, but some close friends have found it very useful.

Wavicle Work begins with a similar attention and loving attunement to your body-mind, and then moves into directly repro-gramming your beliefs and meeting your unconscious needs with unconditional love in order to support your conscious desires. Wavicle Work culminates in the heartfelt acknowledgment of the nature of your devatas as your divine children, made in your image, just as you are an expression of the divine Wholeness itself. When you give your devatas or senses whatever they need on the feeling-level, they manifest that feeling of fullness and completion directly into the physical realm. The tangible results of WW, of experiencing Heaven on Earth, are often swift and wonderful.

Transactional Analysis, Reparenting, and Wavicle Work

In the 1950s Canadian psychiatrist Eric Berne developed Trans-actional Analysis (TA), dividing the personality into Parent, Adult, and Child ego states. In 1964 he wrote the best-selling *Games People Play*, and the TA phrase, "I'm OK, you're OK" became famous.

Transactional Analysis therapist Jacqui Lee Schiff created Reparenting, which involved "decathecting" or erasing a schizophrenic patient's current Parent ego state and recreating a new one. She herself played the part of her many live-in patients' new mother, even putting her patients in diapers, allowing them to breastfeed, and administering spankings and other corporal punishment when she deemed it necessary. She wrote *All My Children* in 1970, and enjoyed a great deal of fame until resigning from the International Transactional Analysis Association in 1978 amidst evidence of severe physical and emotional abuse of patients. She continued practicing overseas however, despite continuing accusations of abuse.

In 1994 the *Transactional Analysis Journal* published Alan Jacobs' seminal article, "Theory as Ideology: Reparenting and Thought Reform," pointing out the potential for abuse of power inherent in the brainwashing nature of Schiff's Reparenting. I have read the book *I'm OK, You're OK* but have not practiced TA or Reparenting, though some close relatives enjoyed it for many years.

While Wavicle Work also repatterns old belief systems by playing the part of an ideal parent to your inner children or thought-wavicles, WW follows a strict script of unconditional love, disallows the physical acting out of issues, and encourages you to do your own restructuring, thus avoiding the potential for misuse or abuse of power by a facilitator. By acknowledging the celestial or divine nature of your wavicles, you may experience not merely healthier parenting, but divinity itself.

Breathwork Techniques and Wavicle Work

After LSD research was banned in the late 1960s, transpersonal psychiatrist Stansilav Grof developed Holotropic Breathwork to access "non-ordinary" states of consciousness and healing through accelerated breathing techniques in conjunction with evocative music. Other elements may include Mandala drawings and focused energy-release work.

In the 1970s and 1980s, Babaji devotees Leonard Orr and Sondra Ray developed Rebirthing-Breathwork, which involves paying attention to the breath and allowing the body to bring long-suppressed traumas – including the birth trauma – to your awareness for integration and healing. Orr and Ray also combined breathwork with reprogramming your beliefs to help you structure physical immortality and abundance.

At about the same time, Dr. Gay and Kathlyn Hendricks developed the similarly body-centered Radiance Breathwork technique which also promotes awareness and integration of deep-seated unconscious material.

I practiced Rebirthing for several years with excellent results. I have read Sondra Ray and Leonard Orr's *Rebirthing in the New Age* (1983), Ray's *The Only Diet There Is* (1987), *Loving Relationships*, *I Deserve Love*, and *Ideal Birth* (all 1995), and Orr's *Breaking the Death Habit: The Science of Everlasting Life* (1998), have met them both, and respect their work.

Wavicle Work's preliminary attention to the breath and body is similar to Rebirthing, and Sondra Ray's affirmations and "payoff technique" –"one of the *great* things about [this problem] is [fill in whatever comes to mind], and I can have that even with [the desired result]" – are priceless for integrating subconscious objections to growth. Their pioneering work in immortality and prosperity is most admirable.

However, Rebirthing is usually rather prolonged and may produce temporary side-effects like yawning and tetany (involuntary muscular tightening). In Rebirthing there is also the possibility of physical abuse; in April 2000, Rebirthing therapists in Denver accidentally killed ten-year-old Candace Newmaker by wrapping her tightly in a flannel blanket and pushing pillows down onto her to simulate a birth experience.

Wavicle Work avoids all physical re-enactments of any trauma. It begins with a few moments of conscious breathwork and unconditional acceptance, then moves into loving dialogue with your body's inner wisdom in order to determine your real needs and thereby quickly and consciously realign and reprogram your old unconscious conditioning. Depending upon your needs, you may reprogram your wavicles to accept and enjoy not only physical immortality and abundance, but absolutely anything else you and they may deeply desire, including a full remembrance and activation of their (and your) own perfect dharma and eternally divine enlightenment here and now. The results can be astonishingly swift and far-reaching.

Ho' oponopono and Wavicle Work

Ho'oponopono, an ancient Hawaiian ritual of forgiveness, reconciliation, and healing, was updated by kahuna healer Morrnah Nalamaku Simeona (1913-1992), who integrated Christian prayer to the Creator and concepts of karma and reincarnation from Eastern philosophies and Edgar Cayce. Her techniques use the three parts of the mind: subconscious (*'Unihipili*), conscious (*'Uhane*), and superconscious (*'Aumakua*) to cut all *aka cords* or emotional attachments, cleanse old errors in thought, word, and deed, and develop a working relationship with the Divinity within.

Morrnah Simeon wrote three textbooks: *Self-Identity through Ho'oponopono (SITH), Basic 1; Basic 2;* and *Basic 3*. She founded Pacifica Seminars in the 1970s and The Foundation of I, Inc. (Freedom of the Cosmos) in 1980, and taught her SITH technique throughout the United States, Asia, and Europe.

Ho'oponopono was further adapted, simplified, and popularized by Morrnah Simeona's former student, Dr. Ihaleakala Hew Len, who with Joe Vitale wrote *Zero Limits: The Secret Hawaiian System for Wealth, Health, Peace, and More* (2007). Over the course of several years Dr. Len had reportedly cured an entire clinic of the criminally insane simply by practicing Ho'oponopono while looking at their files in his office. As currently taught in his book, a practitioner of Ho'oponopono takes full responsibility for everything in his or her reality and heals whatever needs healing by repeating the phrases *"I love you.*

I'm sorry. Please forgive me. Thank you." I have read the book and have occasionally practiced this form of Ho'oponopono.

Much as in Morrnah Simeona's Ho'oponopono, in Wavicle Work you integrate the three forms of mind or soul by connecting the unconditional love of your spirit (superconscious) through your conscious mind directly with your body (via the subconscious). And as in Dr. Len's Ho'oponopono, in Wavicle Work you take full responsibility for unconditionally loving your creation; you may apologize and ask forgiveness for hurting your wavicle, and you take a few simple steps to integrate and heal whoever is suffering in it. Unlike the form of ho'oponopono presented in *Zero Limits*, however, Wavicle Work also specifically fulfills the unmet desires of those wavicles in your creation who are suffering, allowing them to evolve by reminding them of their inherent divinity and thereby enlivening miracles in their world to reflect into yours.

The Work of Byron Katie and Wavicle Work

Perhaps one of the clearest sages now alive, Byron Katie awoke in 1986 by realizing that when she believed her thoughts, she suffered, and when she didn't believe them, she didn't suffer – and that this was a universal truth. She developed a quick, reliable technique to eradicate suffering for everyone. Her books include *Loving What Is: Four Questions That Can Change Your Life*; *I Need Your Love – Is That True? How to Stop Seeking Love, Appreciation, and Approval, and Start Finding Them Instead*; *A Thousand Names for Joy: Living in Harmony with the Way Things Are*; *Question Your Thinking, Change the World: Quotations from Byron Katie*; *Who Would You Be Without Your Story: Dialogues with Byron Katie*; *Tiger, Tiger – Is It True?*, and *Peace in the Present Moment*, co-authored with Eckhart Tolle.

The Work consists of four questions which you apply to any thought creating pain or discomfort: 1) Is it true? 2) Can you absolutely know that it is true? 3) How do you react when you believe that thought? 4) Who would you be without that thought? Follow this with a turn-around, seeing if an opposite thought – switching subject and object, or making it self-referential – is equally true or truer.

The Work shows you that the source of your suffering is not outside of you; but arises from your own thoughts, which are stressful because they resist your own reality with the idea that things "should" be different. The Work quickly shows you the inherent untruth of any belief and the pain of any thought which "lies" or contradicts your reality, and quickly restores you to your original clarity and peaceful innocence.

Byron Katie's Work provides two crucial realizations – that you are not your thoughts, and that your painful thoughts are not real, not true. The result is a liberating relief and often unconditional love. I have read Byron Katie's earlier books, practiced The Work, and watched her practice on others, and I have consistently been impressed and moved by the beautiful work she does.

Wavicle Work effects a similar liberation by localizing the source of your thought within your body, thereby seeing the thought as your child, your own creation, to whom you offer unconditional love and acceptance. From here, Wavicle Work engages in fulfilling your desire completely on your innermost feeling-level by restoring your thought to its divine stature and bringing it home into your own Wholeness.

Emotional Freedom Technique (EFT) and Wavicle Work

Gary Craig drew on Dr. Roger Callahan's Thought Field Therapy (TFT) as well as acupuncture, neuro-linguistic programming, and energy medicine to create the Emotional Freedom Technique (EFT) in 1993. It is informally known as "Tapping," as like TFT it involves tapping on specific meridian points – top of the head, eyebrows, side of the eye, under the eye, under the nose, chin, collarbone, under the arms, and wrists –while also thinking of the problem you wish to address and speaking an affirmation like the phrase, "Even though I have this [problem], I deeply and completely accept myself."

Though I have not practiced this technique, some close friends have for many years, and they have found it beneficial. I believe EFT's "tapping" would ground the awareness in specified areas in the upper part of the body, and the affirmation offers unconditional acceptance (and love) *despite* the issue. Wavicle Work pays attention directly to the affected area(s) throughout the body and affirms unconditional love directly *to* the issue, integrating and healing it very quickly. In WW you also affirm your wavicle's inherent divinity, ask it what it most needs, and give it that, here and now.

Postscript: A Few Testimonials

We have cited various specific experiences with Wavicle Work in their appropriate chapters; here are a few general testimonials:

"Forty-plus years of serious practice of meditation, in this case TM, found its way 30 years ago into supplemental therapies, behavioral, cognitive and Rebirthing. I was led in this direction simply because meditation brought to the surface emotional patterns, but did not, nor was it designed to, heal them completely. An Odyssey of therapy, involving six therapists, including Ellen Maslow, did indeed unearth and untangle triggers that made my personal life a campaign against anxiety and punctuated by bouts of depression.

"Granted, such therapies went a long way to minimize the frequency and depth of these troughs, but endless recycling of the same 'story' left something to be desired. Rebirthing fared quite a bit better, mainly because it was somatically targeted, although much of the syndrome prevailed.

"A nagging question thus remained: Is there ANY method to bring the mind-body circuit into harmony with itself as well as quicken the grounding of higher states of consciousness that I was beginning to stabilize?

"Rory Goff's Wavicle Work appears to answer both parts of this question. It is simple, elegant, and extremely enjoyable to do and has gotten to the point where it occurs almost by itself with just a little attention. Thus far, I have started to experience deep transformations in my relationships, life work, finances, and feeling a loving world cradling me in its everlasting arms. Life is becoming wonderfully magical. Positivity or negativity, the false duality of three-dimensional 'reality,' is becoming the content of a new book of life, whose every sentence speaks of just how the Awakening is, and has been, Always/Already right Now. No hype: this work is the ticket for anyone aware of the paradigm shift of the planet." – P. J.

"Rory's teaching brings the Divine to where it is not. It is body, feeling, healing and spiritual work. By changing the inner, we transform the outer; we create from the Heart. By embracing everything, we experience Unity, Wholeness. We embrace the ugly so it can show its beauty. No teacher gave me such clarity about karma, suffering, evil — I'm forever grateful to Rory for the depth, clarity and transformative power of his teaching." — Marie Lehrer, Founder and President of Rise Africa

"For me, Particle/Wavicle Work is better now than any form of spiritual technique or herbal remedy. We don't learn how to talk to ourselves in this culture! We don't learn how to be our own mothers! Thanks to Rory and Particle Work I am finally mothering myself, at home with myself, keeping myself company. I have had several semi-serious health problems lately, which have come up because of spiritual transition in my life, and nothing has worked for me at this time other than Particle/Wavicle Work. Rory is not a doctor, but he is very good at sensing subtle energy, and teaching us how to give ourselves what we need, and empowering us to realize and use our power for our own good. Hurray for Rory! He is on the forefront of a new field." — H. J.

"I am very thankful! The wavicle work has been helping me take full responsibility for my life's creation. Yes! All mine! The good and not so good! I have healed not only some challenging emotional and relationship issues but some physical pains as well. Within minutes of acknowledging and allowing the resistance within my physiology and giving it love, acceptance and what it needed to be well, the pain dissipated immediately, just like that. This is totally miraculous yet seemed totally simply ordinary, the way pain should be allowed to heal.

"This technique is truly a simple yet profound way to heal any challenge that comes up, whether it be physical, emotional, mental, or spiritual. A tool that was generously given to me and will be useful for the rest of my life. I am grateful. Thank you, Rory." –B. N.

"How do I learn more?"

We would love to show you Wavicle Work in person! Let us know if there is a group in your area who are interested, and we will arrange a seminar for you and/or book individual private sessions.

You may keep up to date on our website at rorygoff.com and waviclework.com. Please email us at rorygoff@hotmail.com, or write to us at:

Rory Goff
P.O. Box 1058
Fairfield, IA 52556